STUDIOS

T A L M A

Also by Angelina Cai:
- *La Santé par la médecine traditionnelle chinoise*, éd. Louise Courteau, Quebec.

Talma Studios International Ltd.
Clifton House, Fitzwilliam St Lower,
Dublin 2 – Ireland
www.talmastudios.com
info@talmastudios.com
Cover Image: © Maor Glam | Dreamstime.com

ISBN : 978-1-913191-12-2

Angelina Jingrui Cai

DEFEATING COVID-19
AND OTHER VIRUSES
WITH TRADITIONAL
CHINESE MEDICINE

TALMA
STUDIOS

Acknowledgements

To my parents, for keeping my grandparent's recipes, to my father who guided me on the road to traditional Chinese medicine,
To my dear son, because he is the model for the photos of acupuncture points in this book and during this busy period of work, he was the one looking after me.
To Patrick Pasin, my publisher, for his precious role,
To Nancy Gomez, for her help in raising awareness of the epidemic,
To Christophe Enderlin, vice-president of the FNMTC, for his constant encouragements,
To Yves Giarmon, president of the FNMTC, for his great trust,
To Yuan Gu, who helped me proofread the texts,
To the couple Zhou and Veronica Antonella for their support and testimony,
To Mr. and Mrs. Liu, Mrs. Xiuping Ye, Mr Zhendi Zhang, Mr. Dominique He, who helped me manage the groups of people who wanted the help of Traditional Chinese Medicine to treat Covid-19,
To Mr. Changhong Wu, who helped me manage the links of the people to be treated,
To Me Jean-Pierre Stouls, for his help and contribution,
To Jacques Van Minden and Anne Lettré for their support.

天降灾难于人间
Unpredictable misfortune on the world

地藏生机救民生
Now Mother Nature is offering us

古来瘟疫知多少
Regardless of the epidemic

谁知解药近咫尺
The cure at hand

2020年 6月9日
于法国 蔡景瑞
Angelina CAI

Foreword

Before the Pandemic

It was my grandfather, Baochi Cai, a renowned traditional Chinese doctor, who introduced me to this age-old knowledge as a teenager: he thought this was the path I should take. Following his advice, I was trained in traditional Chinese medicine (TCM)[1], which I practice mainly in France, where I have been living for many years, and where I am a member of the National Federation of Traditional Chinese Medicine (FNMTC)[2]. Thus, I welcome patients to my practice for all types of health problems.

Given the magnitude of the pandemic, it was almost inevitable that Covid-19 victims would knock on my door, which happened as early as the end of January.

At the time of writing this book, in May, I had dealt with more than a hundred cases, remotely when confinement started, in France, Italy and China, plus about thirty people treated by colleagues, who asked me for my opinion on the prescriptions. This allowed me to widen my field of observation.

Did they all have Covid-19? It is impossible to be sure since there was no test available outside of health care facilities. However, no matter what illness they consulted me for, no one had to be hospitalized afterwards. Consequently, given the results obtained,

---

1. I am a graduate in international acupuncture, and continue to train myself permanently, in particular by following each year in-depth training courses in China.
2. FNMTC website: www.fnmtc.fr.

it seemed necessary to me to share the methods and recipes used, so that they would benefit everyone, especially since the virus has not been definitively eradicated. They will also be beneficial against other lung infections, such as the flu, and even in our everyday life for different ailments.

After the Pandemic

Although this book is intended for individuals as well as professionals, it is not a study in the sense of Western medicine, with randomized, double-blind comparisons, placebo effect measurement, control group, etc. Moreover, it is not a generalized practice in traditional Chinese medicine, where each situation is considered specific and treated as such.

My job is first and foremost to provide care. Still, it is also my duty to communicate results and successes, especially during such a pandemic so that research can progress. Indeed, even if it is **traditional** medicine, it evolves with the energy of the Earth, of nature, of the human being. Knowing the ancient bases, which have proved their worth for more than two millennia, is therefore indispensable, but cannot be sufficient in this world in constant transformation, all the more so when new diseases appear.

My approach is not intended to compare or contrast Western medicine and traditional Chinese medicine, which are both necessary and complementary. However, one of the strengths of TCM is its emphasis on prevention and strengthening the immune system. This is why we focus our actions primarily on the circulation of energy, food, sleep, without which the immune system cannot be healthy.

This book is not a treatise on self-medication or a TCM course: its main objective is to introduce tools and recipes that can help us to live better, by resisting the external aggressions to which we are subjected, including Covid-19. And if it saves even one life, it was worth writing about.

The Yin (阴) and Yang (阳)

According to Chinese tradition, the balance is always in motion between the two opposing, complementary and inseparable forces of Yin and Yang. The Yin, in black, represents the feminine, the Moon, the night, the cold, the darkness, the descending movement, while the white Yang symbolizes the masculine, the Sun, the light, the heat, the action, the momentum, the ascending movement.

Children, both boys and girls, are generally in the abundance of Yang energy because they are always in motion. From their thirties onwards, Yang energy tends to diminish.

Our foods are Yin, Yang or neutral in nature, depending on their color, environment, parts, harvesting season, cooking method.

Let's take the example of the mulberry tree: the leaves are Yin, but those of spring are less Yin than those of winter, the fruits are slightly Yang, the trunk, branches and roots are neutral. Similarly, the flesh of the clementine is Yang, but the fibers are Yin, so you should eat both to balance the energy (the skin is also Yang, hence the interest of the Chenpi).

An imbalance between Yin and Yang energies has consequences, sometimes serious ones, on our health: by being too Yang, we are nervous, anxious, insomniacs, prone to heart attacks, headaches, toothache, sore throat. Being too Yin, we risk depression, low morale, fatigue, poor appearance, loss of appetite, hair, indigestion, swollen belly and oedemes.

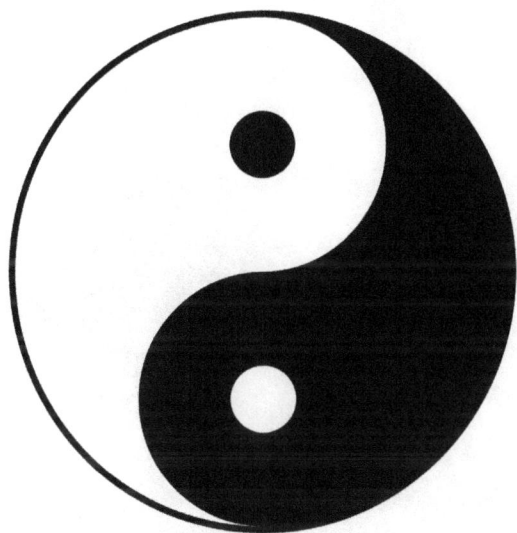

Chapter I

First Encounter
With Covid-19

Back From Wuhan

It is precisely on Sunday, January 25th that I came across the Covid-19 for the first time. The alert to the epidemic has not yet been given in France, but I was approached by a young couple who came back from Wuhan three weeks earlier. They were suffering from a violent cough, day and night, fever—higher in the woman than in the man—sore throat, headaches, loss of appetite, swollen stomach, insomnia and diarrhea.

They had consulted their GP several times without significant improvement. Eventually, their condition worsened, and they decided to call for help from traditional Chinese medicine.

They told me they wear a mask as soon as they leave the house to avoid contaminating those around them. Nevertheless, not being sure of the causes of their symptoms, although everything pointed to the coronavirus that was already wreaking havoc in Wuhan during their stay, I received them at my office on a Sunday, so that they wouldn't cross paths with other patients. Naturally, I followed the necessary protection rules, wearing masks and gloves, and then disinfecting the premises afterwards.

Care, including recipes and ingredients[3], are detailed in the following chapters, but here, in summary, is what I practiced during this first session:

---

3. All products are sold in Asian and specialized supermarkets, often in organic stores and increasingly in other forms of commerce, not to mention internet platforms. Some compositions are even sold ready to use.

– application of suction cups on the Da Zhui and Fei Shu points for the man, Da Zhui and Ding Chuan for the woman, because her condition is more worrying, with difficulties to breathe (Ding Chuan means "stopping the breathing blockage");

– then moxibustion[4] on the same points, to also practice themselves at home every evening for two weeks, to strengthen the Yang energy of the lungs.

Starting with the suction cups allows to rid the body of negative energy quickly, but this technique tends to discharge the energy. At the same time, moxibustion just after will recharge by promoting circulation and helps repair the affected organs.

I recommend the two following recipes for them to prepare themselves:

– an infusion of 50 g of Chinese absinthe (see box A little comparative botany) + 50 g of *Artemisia annua* or annual mugwort + 50 g of *Houttuynia cordata*, also called "Chinese pepper" or "pepper herb," dried, as well as Yu Ping Feng San[5] in the proportions indicated in the box below, to be taken in the morning and evening for seven days;

– an infusion of 50 g of grated ginger with 30 g full-bodied brown sugar[6], to drink in the morning for two weeks.

They bought the ingredients when they left my office and continue the treatment the same evening. They called me the very next day to inform me that their condition was beginning to improve, especially the cough and sore throat, and the fever had already disappeared.

---

4. This technique is presented in Chapter IV. In summary, it consists in heating acupuncture points with a moxa or mugwort stick.

5. Yu Ping Feng San (玉屏風散), literally "jade screen against the wind," is a composition of the Chinese pharmacopoeia which, among other things, tones up vital energy (the Qi) and is mainly used in the case of lung infections.

6. For medicinal recipes, we always use cane sugar, crystallized, brown or full-bodied ("Sha Tang" in Chinese, which means "stimulation of Qi and blood"), never white sugar.

When they came back to my office a week later, they were much better. I recommended that they continue with Yu Ping Feng San for seven more days to strengthen their immune system. At the end of the week, they had no more symptoms and felt cured.

Unusual Combinations
From more than one hundred people who subsequently approached me, the majority could not be accommodated in health facilities because they had conditions ranging from mild to more worrying, but without serious respiratory problems. In the absence of available tests, it was the symptoms, in combinations unlike any other disease (see box), including seasonal influenza, which guided me each time in the diagnosis and solutions to be applied. Patients who had tested positive at the hospital also questioned me.

In summary, my finding is that the symptoms of Covid-19 can be very heterogeneous from one person to another, and even between the elderly, adults, children, women, men, including with disparities between different regions. This may seem surprising, but it is much less so when we know the importance of nutrition on our health.

For example, I observed pronounced differences between patients in France, Italy and China. In addition to apprehending all cases individually, as every doctor must do regardless of their specialty, it became necessary to follow them almost daily, because if the symptoms of Covid-19 vary from one person to another, they can also differ between the day before and the day after, or even disappear before returning a few days later.

Main Symptoms of Covid-19

Here are the first warning signs:
- fever;
- cough;
- aches and pains;
- generalized fatigue;
- shortness of breath;
- thick tongue with a white or yellow coating.

These symptoms are similar to those of the flu. However, some may get worse and progress like this:
- acute respiratory distress;
- acute renal failure;
- multi-visceral failure, which is a condition in which one or more organs deteriorate rapidly.

Other symptoms may appear, such as loss of taste or smell and lack of appetite. There have also been some situations with dizziness and loss of consciousness.

In case of symptoms of respiratory infection (fever, cough, difficulty in breathing), it is recommended :
- to wear a surgical mask and to respect the barrier gestures if you are is in contact with other people;
- use disposable tissues;
- wash your hands frequently.

These are also practices to be adopted for prevention, so even without declared symptoms, especially since Covid-19 may have a long incubation period.

Suppose you have any doubt about having been contaminated. In that case, it is essential to consult a doctor urgently, in order to prevent the deterioration of your condition and also to protect the health of your loved ones.

Remarks

1) In my family of doctors, we are careful not to take the prescriptions for more than seven days, as this can create other imbalances. At the end of this period, we check our health and decide on what to do. Indeed, seven days is usually enough to make significant changes in the body, perhaps not always to remove the root of the disease. Still, the rest of the treatment is then adapted accordingly.

2) For preparations, including infusions, preferably avoid iron or bronze pots, as these materials can interfere and generate side effects, or even alter the effectiveness of the compositions. Instead, choose earthenware, porcelain, glass or stainless steel pots or pans.

3) Most of the treatments presented below can be practiced by everyone, effectively and safely if the rules and recommendations are followed.

A Bit of Comparative Botany

The Artemisia or mugwort type, groups together a large number of plants, whose correspondences and denominations between the Chinese pharmacopoeia and Western botany can generate confusion, which should be cleared up before continuing our presentation.

Thus, when it comes to absinthe, we are not talking about the wormwood or *Artemisia absinthium L.*, used to produce the alcohol of the same name which caused havoc, especially in the 19th century. However, it also belongs to the Artemisia type.

In fact, the one used in the recipes in this book corresponds to 青蒿 (Qinghao), i.e. the *Artemisia annua*, also called "annual wormwood" or "Chinese absinthe." It will therefore appear under the name "absinthe" in the different recipes proposed below.

As for mugwort, it is the species known as "Chinese mugwort," 艾草 (Aicao) or *Artemisia argyi* in western botany.

In summary, we obtain the following taxonomic equivalences:

Absinthe = Chinese absinthe = *Artemisia annua*
= annual mugwort = 青蒿 (Qinghao)

Artemisia = Chinese artemisia = *Artemisia argyi*
= 艾草 (Aicao).

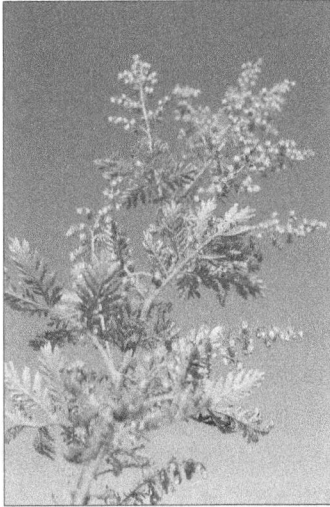

Artemisia annua
/ Chinese Absinthe
/ 青蒿 (Qinghao)
Source: Stefan.lefnaer
/ Commons Wikimedia

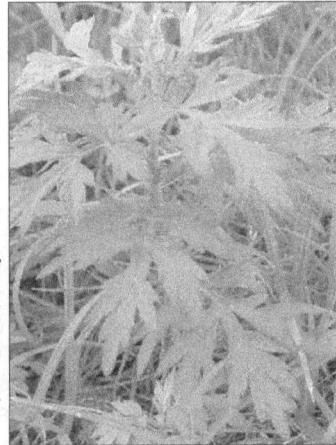

Artemisia argyi
/ Chinese mugwort
/ 艾草 (Aicao)
Source: Commons Wikimedia

Let's remember that a Chinese scientist, Youyou Tu, was awarded the Albert-Lasker Prize for Clinical Medical Research 2011 and the Nobel Prize for Physiology or Medicine 2015 for her work on artemisinin, the active medicinal substance isolated from *Artemisia annua* (青蒿). The medicinal virtues of the latter have been known in China for more than two thousand years. It is used to treat malaria and has saved millions of lives worldwide, particularly in developing countries.

Here, in summary, is how traditional Chinese medicine considers these two plants:

– 青蒿 (*Artemisia annua*) is Yin in nature (see box on Yin and Yang), related to the meridians of the liver and gallbladder.

In addition to its effects against malaria, it is used to regulate the immune system and reduce nervousness. It is also considered antibacterial and anti-cancer.

Although it has been used for two millennia in China, particularly against malaria, it is nevertheless not recommended by the WHO and is banned in some countries.

– 艾草 (Chinese mugwort) is of a warm nature, linked to the meridians of the liver, spleen and kidneys.

It is known to promote the circulation of Qi or "vital energy," strengthen the immune system, remove moisture from the body, soothe coughs, relieve asthma, reduce phlegm, relax and be anti-allergenic and antibacterial.

Yu Ping Feng San (玉屏风散)

It was as early as January 20th, 2020 that I proposed this formula for prevention, to be taken for seven days in the mornings and evenings, to strengthen the immune system and better defend oneself against the coming pandemic. Of the approximately 300 people who confirmed that they had taken it, none of them subsequently reported to me that they had been affected by Covid-19. This is not evidence, nor is it a surprise.

I subsequently recommended it to the hundred or so people who were affected, in addition to the other solutions explained below.

However, just like medicines, the plants in the Chinese pharmacopoeia cannot be taken without professional advice. Yu Ping Feng San is an excellent example. Here is the original recipe:

– 60 g of astragalus root (黄芪), to strengthen the Qi or vital energy;

– 60 g of atractyl root or rhizome (白术), to boost the Yang energy of the spleen;

– 30 g *Saposhnikoviae Radix* (防风), for its protective role.

To reduce the risk of possible side effects, it should be limited to a maximum of seven days and, according to my research and experience, the proportions should be reduced as such:

– 40 g of talus root;

– 40 g of atractyl rhizome;

– 20 g of *Saposhnikoviae Radix*.

I add 20 g of Poria (茯苓, Fu Ling)[7] and licorice stick between 5 to 8 g (do not exceed this dose for this recipe, unless otherwise advised by a professional), for its multiple and precious properties: it strengthens the spleen and kidneys; it is a disinfectant of the pulmonary tract, which soothes coughs and removes mucus; it is indispensable in most "magic potions," as it allows for better results, especially in case of a virus, therefore with Covid-19.

This composition is cautious compared to the original version. Still, it seems to be more balanced in Yin and Yang energy, so that a more significant number of people can use it, especially to prevent or treat symptoms of Covid-19, flu and other lung inflammations, asthma and airway blockages. For children under 12 years of age, doses should be halved.

In general, this preparation should be taken in the morning and evening for seven days. Boil the ingredients in five bowls of water, then reduce to the equivalent of one bowl over low heat. You can drink it.

Don't throw away the plants that remain at the bottom of the pot: reboil five bowls according to the same principle for the evening potion. The next day, however, take new ingredients.

Caution: Yu Ping Feng San remains a medicinal composition, which needs to be prescribed by professionals of traditional medicine and not to be self-prescribed.

And if prevention does not work, do not wait to consult your doctor.

---

7. This is a mushroom that has been used for a long time in TCM, mainly as a fortifier, but also to give balance.

No Social Networking Care!
Never take any medication or treatment without consulting a doctor. The same is true in traditional Chinese medicine. For example, on March 5th, I received a message from a friend who had found a Chinese pharmacopoeia recipe on a WeChat group, the well-known Chinese messaging service. The result is that, for the past eight days, the whole family had been suffering from diarrhea, including her six-month-old daughter, whom she was breastfeeding.

I asked her why she took the risk of using a recipe without first seeking advice from a medical professional? Unsurprisingly, she confirms that fear guided her, and since it was only herbal, it couldn't hurt them. Of course, it could! It is imperative not to consume any given plant at any given time for any given symptom(s), and not to assemble them either without a thorough knowledge of the possible combinations, because some plants taken at the same time can produce toxic effects that they do not have when consumed separately.

In addition, given their condition, my friend asked the person who had published this recipe whether their diarrhea was normal. She was told that yes, it even proved that the body was detoxifying. Again, it doesn't work that way, and that is a very serious statement. Indeed, I cannot imagine, after eight days of diarrhea, what state their bodies and immune systems were in? It is evident that if one of their relatives had started to show the symptoms of Covid-19, it would have been almost impossible to escape it, and even to resist a simple cold, let alone flu.

So I recommended:

– to stop the diarrhea: Immediately a large bowl of infusion of grated ginger and brown sugar, to be taken every morning for three days - except for the baby, who would benefit from the mother's milk;

– to strengthen the energy of the lungs: an infusion of wormwood, to be drunk in the morning and evening during the next three days, after diarrhea has disappeared;

– to strengthen the immune system, from the first day and for a week: a moxa on the belly once a day for everyone, including the baby, who had begun to lose its appetite.

My friend called me at the end of the week to let me know that they were cured and to thank me.

Although traditional Chinese medicine played a significant role in defeating this coronavirus in China, it was scary to read daily on social media about new supposedly miraculous recipes being marketed at often exorbitant prices by unscrupulous sellers masquerading as doctors of traditional Chinese medicine. Fear should not guide us, because the "medicine" may be worse than the ache. So be careful and vigilant, your health and that of your loved ones is at stake.

Sharing of Information
In response to these dangerous, even criminal acts, I began disseminating on social media in France and China information on what Covid-19 is from the point of view of traditional Chinese medicine, with the means of prevention and care, recommendations for daily life, particularly concerning diet and physical exercise, what to do if the first symptoms appear, the role of vitamins, etc. Every day, I gave nearly three hours of live lectures, with up to 2,000

participants, answering their many questions. As a result, most if not all of them stopped blindly shopping on the internet. Also, I was called upon for private and remote care sessions, many of which couldn't be accommodated by health facilities, usually because their conditions were not considered severe enough.

My period of confinement suddenly became overloaded: (volunteer) care during the day, conferences and exchanges in the evening. I quickly exceeded the number of one hundred patients that I had to care for. I am not claiming that this is a broad basis for analysis, but action is needed, sometimes in the face of situations of medical distress. The results allowed me to confirm my diagnoses and validate the care to be provided, similar to the ones I already used, especially in cases of lung infection. The information was spreading, Chinese media even interviewed me on two topics:
– traditional Chinese medicine in the face of the epidemic;
– its place in Western medicine.

Straight From the Doctors in Wuhan

On April 20th, I participated in an online conference with Chinese doctors, several of whom belong to the Tang Po Xue[8] group, on the front lines of medical interventions in Wuhan. The founder and leader of this volunteer group, Dr. Wu, Director of the Department of Lung Diseases at Xianning[9] Chinese Medicine Hospital, in the Hubei province, the region most affected by Covid-19, represents like me the fourth generation of a line of traditional doctors. His team, created three years ago, is composed of about two hundred traditional doctors known in China for their unique acupuncture methods and knowledge of TCM.

---

8. The name Tang Po Xue comes from a proverb in acupuncture: "Treating a disease effectively and quickly is like melting snow with warm water."
9. Capital city of south-eastern Hubei with more than 2.5 million inhabitants.

As soon as the epidemic arrived, they volunteered to join the medical teams mobilized in Wuhan and other cities in the province. They treated nearly five hundred patients, including about forty severe or critical cases. All those who followed the prescriptions recovered—there were a few cases, unfortunately, who could not access the prescribed pharmacopoeia or follow the recommended treatment. The doctors of the Tang Po Xue group also carried out remote interventions in about ten other countries (Germany, Spain, France, the Netherlands, the United Kingdom, Chile, Turkey, Nepal, the United States and Canada), with similar results.

In medicine in general and in our practice in particular, the state of the tongue is a valuable indicator (see Appendix 1). The pulse is another, but in periods of confinement, it is possible to send pictures of the tongue, not the pulse. Since my colleagues found, for the majority of patients (in China), that their tongue was yellow or abnormally red and dry, most of them classified the epidemic in 温病 (Wēn Bîng), i.e. as "lukewarm epidemic disease" and in 湿温 (Shī Wen), "wet and lukewarm disease." As a result, they opted for the techniques of Ye Tianshi, the famous 18th-century Chinese physician (see *Chapter II*), which consists of treating with plants of a Yin nature.

One of the explanations would come from the fact that the region of Wuhan has a humid climate; therefore the cuisine there is too spicy to eliminate the excess moisture produced in the body by the climatic conditions. In fact, I remember my last training there, when I couldn't eat their dishes even though I asked the chef not to add any chilli or hot sauce. It was still too spicy for me. The next few days, I only ate white rice with a little soy sauce and fruit—luckily their fruits are not spicy.

According to the principles of traditional Chinese medicine, despite the humidity of the climate, spicy food generates, in the long run, an overabundance of Yang energy, which takes Yin energy away from the body, creating a Yin deficiency and thus an imbalance. Without embarking on a fictional scenario, it is legitimate to wonder whether the epidemic would have broken out so virulently in a region with less humidity and a more balanced diet between Yin and Yang?

At this conference, I could share my observations on patients not living in Wuhan or its region with the Tang Po Xue group. In my opinion, we cannot determine whether Covid-19 is a disease in 温疫 (Wēn Yî, "lukewarm epidemic disease") or 寒疫 (Han Yî, "epidemic cold disease"). Indeed, out of the hundred or so patients that I followed, their tongue was, contrary to what my colleagues in Wuhan found, mostly pale in color, with a thick but white layer, or even a light yellow layer on top of a thick white layer for some.

On the other hand, as in Wuhan, I had the case of a woman with a thick yellow tongue, although she lived in France. Her condition was quite serious: she could hardly breathe at night, had lost her sense of taste and smell, coughed a lot, had a persistent fever, and even traces of blood in her mucus. In addition, she was so exhausted that she couldn't even make it down the stairs. Not being able to be hospitalized, she asked me for help.

To suppress the fever, I used a recipe of my grandmother, Zhefei Dai, based on garlic, ginger and chives (see below), and, for the other symptoms, I recommended a solution similar to the one for the Wuhan couple, with an infusion composed of 50 g of mugwort + 50 g of dried *Houttuynia cordata* + Yu Ping Feng San in the proportions indicated in the box, to be taken during seven days morning and evening.

At the end of the week, I recommended drinking white radish soup with honey twice a day for seven days, alternating every other day with an infusion of dried mandarin peel (called "Chenpi" — it will be specified below what it is, as for each recipe and ingredient) with licorice stick.

I also recommended it from the beginning:

– to eat dandelions, in salad or stir-fry, apple and dried figs (it was not yet the season for fresh figs);

– to practice moxibustion on Da Zhui, Fei Shu and Ding Chuan points, morning and evening for seven days;

– to take foot baths with 50 g of moxa leaves and ten slices of ginger before going to sleep.

She followed this program to the letter, with the following results: the disappearance of the fever from the second day; progressive improvement of the cough and breathing returned to normal by the end of the first week, with the return of taste and smell and the disappearance of the feeling of tiredness. Moreover, she testified to Chinese journalists about the effectiveness of my recommendations.

At the end of the conference with the Chinese doctors, we decided to set up an exchange group, to continue sharing our methods and results, which is usual in our field.

Note: I followed almost daily the evolution of the people who consulted me, especially the most worrying cases that could not be treated in hospital. For example, I asked them to send me daily pictures of their tongues. In the serious case of the lady above, it gradually began to change color, and the layer became thinner and thinner until it disappeared. So when she was healed, her tongue had turned pink again, and there was no more thick layer.

Four Examples

In order to arrive at solutions without delay, I do not wish to multiply the presentation of cases that I have had to deal with. However, the following four examples are representative of the types of situations encountered and allow us to orient our reflection on prevention.

It should be noted that systematically, unless otherwise specified, the recommendation is for one week. It will not be repeated each time.

1) The L family.[10]

In all countries, it has been observed that Covid-19 can have a long incubation period, up to 14 days, and is highly contagious: this means that when one member of a family catches it, it is almost inevitable that everyone will get it, although it may not be triggered, depending on their health and immune system.

In this way, Mrs. L., whose husband had just been tested positive to Covid-19 and brought urgently to the hospital by an ambulance, called me on April 15th. Mrs L., her twenty-year-old son and her eighteen-year-old daughter, also showed symptoms, but at a less worrying level than Mr L. Of the three, Mrs L. is, however, the most affected: she has lost her sense of smell and appetite, her tongue is thick with a yellow coating, she coughs day and night and suffers from throat pain, fever and diarrhea. In addition, she has insomnia, which weakens her further and thus also reduces her ability to resist the disease.

My advice to her is:

– the same infusion recipe as above, based on wormwood, mugwort and Yu Ping Feng San for a week;

– then, to remove the persistent yellow mucus: for three days, some pear soup with white cane sugar;

10. Even though the patients cited in this book have authorized me to use their name, and some of them even gave interviews where they testify of my interventions and their results, I do not use their name out of respect for the medical secret.

– and afterwards, dried mandarin peel (Chenpi) and licorice sticks for three days also.

She also uses the Guasha technique twice in three days (see *Chapter IV*).

In terms of food, I recommend millet, dandelions, in salads or stir-fries, apples and dried figs.

Results: fever falls, and diarrhea stops the next day, cough improves and sore throat disappears in three days, breathing and sense of smell return to normal after the first week. Her appetite returns with the return of her husband, and sleep does too with the practice of foot baths every night, which she continues since she was cured.

As for the children, I advise drinking Yu Ping Feng San morning and evening for three days, then infusion of Chenpi + liquorice morning, noon and evening for a week, as both have a slightly thick white tongue. They also practice two sessions of Guasha.

As a result, the cough and sore throat disappear for good after a week, at the end of which they no longer have any symptom.

2) Mrs. A.

On May 6th, a lyric solo artist in France contacted me and described her condition in such words:

> I had the first symptoms of Covid on March 15th. The diagnosis is 100% sure since I did a lung scan which marks the stigmata of the virus.
>
> However, almost two months later, I am still experiencing the first signs of breathing difficulties, which my pulmonologist treats as asthma. I still haven't regained my sense of taste and smell.

The problem is that my job requires my lungs. The voice is there, but it's the lungs that are weak.

So there is no doubt about the disease since this patient was diagnosed and treated at the hospital. However, after-effects persist, with significant professional consequences, since she is no longer able to practice her profession almost two months after the beginning of the disease.

My first question is about what antibiotic(s) she took. They can indeed modify the immune system and, by repercussion, the recommendations of traditional Chinese medicine.

First azithromycin, then Clamoxyl, following a dental infection, and metronizadole when the tooth became superinfected.

I then questioned her in detail about her symptoms and her body's reactions and asked for a picture of her tongue. Upon receipt, I can diagnose that Mrs. A. had low energy in her lungs and kidneys, which meant that there was still moisture and mucus to be removed.

Her breathing difficulties made it hard for her to fall asleep. The priority, of course, was to boost the immune system, and the most effective and natural way to do this was to restore sleep first. I recommend a foot bath with about ten slices of ginger for twenty minutes before going to bed.

I also suggested drinking the following infusion morning and evening for seven days: Absinthe (20 g) + Mugwort (20 g) + Yu Ping Fen San + Mandarin fiber (20 g) + Mulberry leaf (20 g); and practicing moxibustion on Da Zhui, Fei Shu and Ding Chuan points twice a day, morning and evening.

On May 7th, that is to say, the very next day, she sent me the following message:

I slept well last night. Efficient ginger foot bath! I didn't take any Xanax.

I also advised her if she could afford it, to make millet soup and add brown sugar to give her energy. In the following days, she confirmed to me the benefits she felt in terms of breathing and sleep. She also told me that she mentioned my treatment to a news agency that came to interview her.

Four days later, on May 11th, she asked me the following questions:

Is it normal that I'm disgusted by the sweetness of herbal tea?

I answered:

Congratulations, you got your taste back!

The next day, the sense of smell also came back:

Because I could smell the soup cooking this morning—a terrible smell and a miracle, thank you !!!

In short, she regained her taste and smell by following these recipes for five to six days, whereas they had been lost for two months with the onset of the disease. If some people prefer to think that this is only a placebo effect, it proves that humans are powerful. Who can really doubt it? This is illustrated by the third case below.

Before presenting it, here is the end of the recommendations for Mrs. A., who sent me two pictures of her tongue on May 13th. They showed that she was cured. Nevertheless, to better tone the energy of her lungs, I recommended that she should drink without

moderation for two weeks and alternating every three days the following infusions:
– mint (fresh) + honey;
– lemongrass;
– thyme + verbena.

Coughing causes a lack of Yin energy in the lungs. It is, therefore, preferable to start with the infusion mint + honey, because the whole is rather Yin, which allows to rehydrate them at first. Then, the lemongrass is slightly Yang, therefore effective to re-energize the lungs and disinfect them thoroughly. Finally, the thyme + verbena infusion in the third stage being balanced in Yin and Yang, it rebuilds the energy of the other organs impacted by the weakness of the lungs (we will come back to this point).

As I also notice a slight form of stress, even anxiety, I advise her to take care of her liver, particularly by following these recommendations:
– eating artichokes, arugula, dandelions, calf's liver.
– drinking infusions of dried rose petals (seven buds in a cup) + one or two sticks of dried licorice + one or two slices of dried hawthorn. In addition, this infusion is considered to have rejuvenating, beautifying and slimming effects. It goes to show how valuable is the recipe.

And, whenever possible, continuing foot baths and moxibustion on Da Zhui, Fei Shu and Ding Chuan point twice a day, morning and evening.

On May 26th, Mrs. A. sent me the results of her chest CT scan:

Indication
Control of a Covid-19 infection in March (rare frosted glass

opacities, with nodular appearance, involving less than 10% of lung volume).

(…)

Conclusion:

CT normalization. No abnormalities.

She is therefore definitively cured and sent me a final test report, which concluded: "Presence of anti-Sars-CoV2 (Covid-19) antibodies." There is thus no doubt about the disease that affected her and, moreover, she generated antibodies.

3) The E family.

The story of this Chinese family, which was introduced to me by a friend, touches me particularly. For one week, the father had had a fever, around 38 °C, kept coughing and had lost his appetite. His wife had just started coughing, but had also lost her appetite and could no longer sleep. As for the two children, they showed a slight fever, without any other symptoms.

They called the paramedics, who deemed their condition insufficiently alarming at a time when hospitals were increasingly saturated, and redirected them to their doctor. He recommended Paracetamol.

After a week, there was no improvement, and the fear and anxiety had become more and more present.

When they contacted me, I asked them to answer my questionnaire of about twenty questions and, of course, to send me pictures of their tongues.

Mr E.'s case was the most serious. Here were my recommendations for him:

– my grandmother's herbal tea recipe (garlic + ginger + chives) to remove the fever;

– moxibustion on Da Zhui, Fei Shu and Ding Chuan points twice a day, morning and evening.

Then, as soon as the fever was gone, i.e. two days later, take an infusion of 20 g of Chinese mugwort (艾叶) + Yu Ping Fen San + tangerine fiber (30 g) + mulberry leaf (30 g), for seven days morning and evening.

For Mrs. E.:

– foot baths with about 10 slices of ginger + about 50 g of mulberry leaves;

– Yu Pin Feng San;

– moxibustion on Da Zhui, Fei Shu and Ding Chuan points, twice a day, morning and evening, as for most other patients.

As for the children:

– my grandmother's recipe for removing fever;

– then the same infusions as for Mrs. A., to be taken for a week, alternating: (fresh) mint with honey/lemongrass/thyme + verbena.

My advice reassured Mrs E., but a problem came up: they live more than 300 km from Paris, which makes it challenging to buy the necessary plants. Of course, shipping by post or express services are possible, but the delivery time can be long, so she didn't know when the family would be able to start the recommendations.

That same evening, around 7:00 p.m., I received a call from a man. He was about seventy years old, he was the father of Mrs. E., and wanted to see me with the plants he managed to find in Paris during the day so that I could confirm to him that they are indeed the ones I indicated.

Mrs E. told me later that her father had been running all day through Paris looking for the ingredients, and that after making the detour to see me, he immediately left to join them by car, more than 300 km away. When he arrived, he put his purchases in front of their door, without being able to kiss them or even enter, so as not to risk being contaminated, and drove off again. In the end, he drove nearly 700 km during the night, before being back home in the early morning.

The family was cured a week later.

I also advised them to sunbathe between 10 a.m. and 12 p.m. and then between 3 p.m. and 5 p.m., especially Mr E. Indeed, the sun is natural Yang energy, and it's free! It is recommended to put the back facing the sun to capture Yang energy, rather than the belly, which captures the Yin energy of the Moon. Please also note that the duration and times of exposure to the sun vary according to the seasons and locations. For example, in France, you should avoid choosing between 12:00 and 2:00 p.m. in the summer. For China, it is different.

Every time I think of this father and this family, tears come to my eyes. It's amazing what love can make people do.

4) Mrs. S.

Before becoming a liberal nurse, she worked at the American Hospital in Paris. I have been following her for a long time, and she recommended me to her family and friends, who consult me regularly. She pays a lot of attention to my advice, especially for daily nutrition because, since she started putting them into practice, she has been feeling fit, has regained her energy as well as a good look, has no longer had insomnia, migraine, menstrual pain or inflammation. She has even lost five kilos and is back to being the sweet, smiling woman her relatives knew.

She is proof that traditional Chinese medicine is not a miracle, but a daily practice offered to everyone. It was her evolution that convinced those around her to come and see me.

On March 24th, she began to show the now well-known symptoms of dry cough, sore throat, loss of smell and taste. She was worried, especially since her job as a caretaker exposed her to the risk of Covid-19. A test confirmed that she was positive. She called the paramedics, who recommended that she stayed home and took Paracetamol.

Her situation did not improve, on the contrary, and her breathing became more and more difficult, with increases in anxiety and stress. That is why she decided to call me. After studying the photos of her tongue and her answers to my questionnaire, I recommended her:

– moxibustion twice a day on the points already mentioned above (Da Zhui, Fei Shu and Ding Chuan);

– a large bowl of ginger infusion with brown sugar;

– in the evening: eat raw white radish head, and take a foot bath with 50 g of dried wormwood leaves + 50 g of dried safflower flower + ten slices of ginger ;

– during the day: drink soup with the remaining (boiled) white radish and honey, as well as thick millet soup;

– and, specifically for a sore throat, to include dandelions with roots at lunch, alternating the preparations: in a salad, mixed with rocket leaves; in a soup, with three heads of garlic and coriander; in a drink, with 50 g of liquorice + 50 g of Chenpi ;

– and, if possible, warming her back in the sun every morning between 10 a.m. and 12, then from 3 p.m. to 5 p.m., to absorb Yang energy, as in the case of the E family.

Symptoms quickly disappeared, and a week later, taste and smell returned.

Then, to continue to boost her energy, I recommend that she continued moxibustion on the navel on the Shen Que point (神阙) and/or on the back, on the other side of the navel, on Ming Men (命门), and drink white mushroom soup (20 g) + lotus seeds (20 g) + *Atractylodes macrocephala* Bai Zhu (20 g)[11] + *Poria Fuling* (20 g) + *Semem Euryale's Qianshi* (20 g), once a day for three days, during snack time (although it has a sweet taste and is considered a dessert, it is preferable to consume this soup outside of meals; otherwise it loses its effectiveness).

Mrs. S. quickly regained her full fitness and her activity as a nurse.

After Confinement

When my office reopened at the beginning of June, four people came to see me after being ill with Covid-19, two of whom tested positive and two of whom were untested but showed symptoms of the epidemic. Although they had been affected for more than three

---

11. Chinese medicinal plant, as well as the following two ingredients

months, none of them had yet recovered to their previous state of health. These cases are significant because they are evident that we must remain vigilant about recovery, but that TCM solutions continue to work in the post-pandemic period.

Case 1: Mrs. C., 42 years old, tested positive in February, with all the symptoms we now know well: fever, difficulty breathing, cough, diarrhea, loss of taste and smell. She took Paracetamol on the recommendation of her GP, and got over it, but she still felt exhausted, with migraines and still had difficulty breathing, especially when going up and downstairs.

I started by putting the suction cups on Da Zhui, a Fei Shu point and a Ding Chuan point to help her get rid of the "negativity" that stayed in her lungs. Then, on the two Shen Shu points, because once the Covid-19 has entered the body, it contaminates not only the lungs but also the kidneys, which must be treated: they are considered the root of the organs.

After the suction cups: moxibustion on the same points so that Mrs. C. recovered energy, and then acupuncture to promote circulation.

At the end of the session, she felt that her energy returned and breathing improved.

As her tongue was slightly swollen, with a rather thick yellow layer at the base of the tongue, which corresponds to the kidney area, I recommend the following infusion, to be taken for seven days morning and evening: 50 g of *Artemisia annua* / Chinese wormwood + 10 g of tangerine fiber + 30 g of mulberry leaf + 20 g of Chenpi + 10 g of liquorice + Yu Ping Feng San.

Cases 2 and 3: Mrs. Y., 58 years old, and Mrs. S., 65 years old, had symptoms of Covid-19, but they were not tested and had taken Paracetamol. Given the condition of their tongues during the consultation, similar to that of Mrs C., I proceeded in the same way, with the same results at the end of the session.

Case 4: Mr. R., 57 years old, is a singer and visited me on the advice of a friend, whom I took care of remotely. Tested positive at the beginning of March, he then presented the same symptoms as Mrs C. and had taken Paracetamol on the recommendation of his general practitioner.

Tested again at the end of April, this time he turned out to be negative. During May, he nevertheless felt that the virus is waking up: he has trouble breathing again, his energy was "flat," his lungs were increasingly "blocked," he lost his appetite, insomnia returned, and he could no longer sing. There were also symptoms that I hadn't seen in other cases of coronavirus: knee pain and memory problems. His condition reinforced my observations that Covid-19 does not only affect the lungs and that we absolutely must look at the other organs.

With his pulse, I see, indeed, the weakness of his energy in the heart, liver, lungs and kidneys, with water retention in the spleen. Therefore, we start with the suction cups on Da Zhui, a Fei Shu point, a Ding Chuan point and the two Shen Shu points. The treatments are similar to those of Mrs. C.: after the suction cups, moxibustion on the same points to raise and tone the energy, with the addition of Pi Shu, Gan Shu and Ming Men, followed by acupuncture to promote circulation.

After the session, he is delighted that his knee pain has already disappeared and his breathing is improving. This is what he described feeling during the acupuncture part:

> Warm energy is flowing back into my body; the feeling of coldness is gone, especially in my hands and feet.

Its tongue had a white layer covered with a light yellow layer, so I recommend the following infusion, to be taken for seven days morning and evening: 30 g of *Artemisia annua* / Chinese wormwood (青蒿) + 30 g of Chinese wormwood (艾叶) + 10 g of tangerine fibre + 30 g of mulberry leaf + 20 g of Chenpi + 10 g of liquorice + Yu Ping Feng San.

I also recommended a foot bath with a dozen slices of ginger every evening to chase away insomnia and stimulate energy in the kidneys. Indeed, warming the feet makes the energy of the kidneys circulate and promotes circulation throughout the lower part of the body, which helps us to relax. In traditional Chinese medicine, the feet are considered the root of the body, and the kidneys the root of the organs.

Two Complementary Systems

In China, traditional medicine and western medicine, with the use of chemical drugs, are considered complementary, and the two systems can coexist in the same hospital, the priority being the health of the patient, and therefore the choice of the best solution for him or her.[12]

Having knowledge of Chinese medicines and having had my first experiences with Covid-19, I made a request for donations of Chinese medicines to Mr. Li, the representative in France of the public interest foundation International Education Center (全景公益基金会).

With his support, the foundation he represents and the National Administration of Traditional Chinese Medicine (中国中医药管理局) agreed to supply us with Chinese patented pharmaceutical drugs free of charge, but it was impossible to receive them, due to the required level of import licenses and of the CE standard.

Eventually, they sent us about 200 kg of medicinal plants, which were distributed as soon as they were received, i.e. as of April 8th (the epidemic greatly slowed down the logistics and the arrival of the plants).

In the meantime, a large number of patients had been able to obtain them in specialized shops or to have them sent by their families in China.

---

12. "Across the country, more than 92% of Chinese Covid-19 patients have been treated with TCM alone or in combination with Western therapies." *Wikipedia's Culture of Editorial Chaos and Malice*, Richard Gale and Dr. Gary Null, Global Research, June 19th, 2020.

Chapter II

Sources and Research

Multiple Practices

With the examples of the previous chapter, those who are not familiar with traditional Chinese medicine have noticed that it uses different techniques, which we can summarize in the following non-exhaustive way: pharmacopoeia and herbal medicine, dietetics, acupuncture, moxibustion, energetic exercises and massages, the application of suction cups, Gua Sha. We will come back in more detail below on some of these techniques, at least those that have proven to be effective in overcoming Covid-19.

First Founding Principles

Anyone can be affected by this virus, but traditional Chinese medicine considers that people with a balance of Yin and Yang energy will resist better, or even be affected little or not at all because their immune system will be up to the task of defending them from such attacks.

Secondly, TCM treats each situation individually and does not offer a generalized response, such as a universal drug. In China, for example, the treatment will depend on the province or region, i.e. its cuisine, climate conditions, etc. As a result, I do not give the same recommendations to my patients depending on whether they live in France, Italy, Morocco or China, on the one hand, and the symptoms they present, on the other hand, even if the diagnosis indicates the same disease. Of course, there is a common basis and common aspects, as we have seen in the examples mentioned above, but they are always assessed and treated on a case-by-case basis. Should I have had to deal with patients in sub-Saharan Africa or Northern Europe, the recommendations would probably still have been different. This is actually what the book of the mythical Yellow Emperor, the *Huangdi Nei Jing* (黄帝内经)[13], expresses:

中医是因地制宜，因时制宜，因人制宜的，

which means:

> Chinese medicine adapts to local conditions, adapts to the moment and adapts to the people.

Consequently, the first recommendation of Traditional Chinese Medicine in the face of the coronavirus epidemic is to strengthen our immune system, i.e. "the protective/defensive layer" (卫气, Wei Qi). This consists first of all in balancing our Yin and Yang energies, to allow us to be healthy: prevention is the key. Solutions come later when illness strikes.

Nevertheless, in the case of the Covid-19, do not hesitate to call the services which will be able to bring you the help you need. If, afterwards, although it is necessary, the hospital cannot take you in, note these points: stay at home in a quiet place, drink lukewarm water, i.e. water brought to boiling point and cooled down to around 40 to 50 °C, as it allows us to breathe better than cold water which makes blockages stagnate. Also follow a light diet, with less fat and sugar, which will have a positive effect on symptoms related to Covid-19, colds, flu, fever—for example, if a child coughs, it is best to avoid giving him or her French fries. Don't take any "advice" or even antibiotics that you

---

13. The Huangdi Nei Jing (黄帝内经) or *Internal Classic of the Yellow Emperor* is the oldest work of traditional Chinese medicine. Huangdi, also known in the West as the Yellow Emperor, was a mythical civilizing ruler who is considered the father of China. He would have reigned in the 3rd millennium BC.

may have found on social networks without first seeking a doctor's advice—your health is at stake, as we've already explained.

Before presenting several natural solutions, especially in terms of nutrition, to help us increase our energy and strengthen our immune system, let's introduce synthetically the main sources of traditional Chinese medicine and those I rely on, especially when doctors in my family have developed them—I have actually quoted several times my grandmother's recipes.

The Ancient Masters
First of all, I used the knowledge developed by Zhang Zhongjing (张仲景), a famous master of traditional Chinese medicine. The dates of his birth and death are not known with certainty, but it is estimated that he lived between 150 and 219, i.e. at the end of the Han Dynasty, which ruled China from 206 BC to 220 AD.

His essential book, the *Shanghan Zabing Lun* (伤寒杂病论), which can be translated as the Treatise on Cold Pathologies and Other Diseases, was lost during the wars of the Three Kingdoms period (220-280), but was later reconstructed in two books by different physicians :

– the *Shang Han Lun* (伤寒论) or *Treatise on Cold Damage Diseases*, a book focused on how to treat epidemic infectious diseases causing widespread fevers in his time, and

– the *Jingui Yaolue* (金匮要略) or *Essential Prescriptions from the Golden Cabinet*, a collection of various clinical experiences on internal diseases.

Regularly updated up to the modern era, it has become a classic of traditional Chinese medicine and remains one of the most influential works in the field of health.

From the Yuan (1279-1368) and Ming (1368-1644) dynasties, Zhang Zhongjing was even considered a "medical saint." In addition to the principle of differentiation and treatment of the syndrome that he established, which constitutes the basis and soul of the clinical practice of TCM, he developed numerous dosage forms and prescriptions that have proven their effectiveness for two millennia.

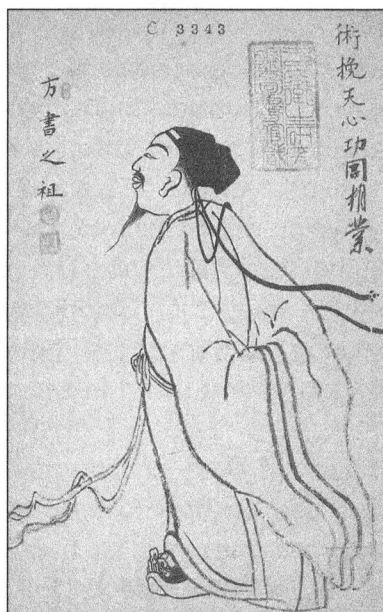

Zhang Zhongjing
Source: Wellcome Images / Wikimedia Commons

Next, I worked from the work of Ye Tianshi (葉天士), born into a family of doctors (1667-1747). His grandfather Ye Shi and his father Ye Zhaocai were exceptionally competent in the field of pediatrics. Ye Tianshi began learning medicine at the age of twelve. A contemporary minister, who wrote a biography of his life, said that everyone knew his works, "even the peddler." He is known not only for his medical skills but also for his mastery of Fengshui techniques.

His work is still relevant today, including in the case of coronavirus, as Ye Tianshi is considered the best source for the treatment of epidemic diseases, as well as malaria and rashes. Incidentally, he was the first in China to discover scarlet fever.

His book *Wenre Lun* (温热论), or *Discussion of Warm Diseases*, was published in 1746, shortly before his death.

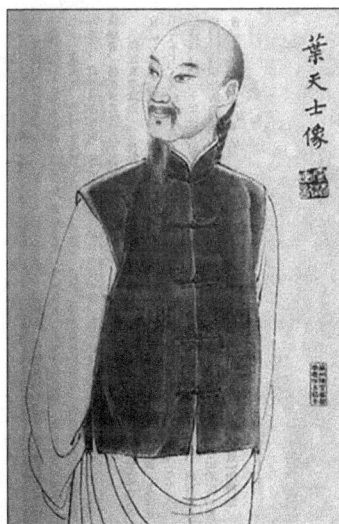

Ye Tianshi
Source: Wikimedia Commons

Family Sources

I mentioned my grandfather, who was a great traditional Chinese doctor, but so was my grandmother, whose recipes I use a lot. She was trained in both western medicine, with a specialization in dermatology, and traditional Chinese medicine. Her father was also a western and traditional Chinese doctor who studied medicine in France. When he returned to China, he practiced his profession and, in addition, was appointed prefect of his province.

My patients benefit from their research, which I am also pursuing because nature and living beings are continually evolving. I began to study the question of Covid-19 as early as January because it seemed apparent that the epidemic would become worldwide (I even sent a warning letter to the French Ministry of Health on February 10th, including proposals for solutions to be implemented, for instance at Charles-de-Gaulle airport).

The first point of my research focused on the analysis of the symptoms, through the files communicated by the doctors in China. I also exchanged with the students of my father, also a doctor, especially with one of them, as he helped teams of caretakers on prevention issues. He shared their experiences, the plants they used, the advances, the failures. I also participated with them in the analyses. Then, I took all the plants and recipes that had proved their effectiveness, which I selected and adapted according to the environment of France and the countries where I usually intervene.

This way, when the couple who returned from Wuhan came to consult me at the end of January, I already knew the solutions to be implemented. Their rapid recovery gave me even more confidence, which was later reinforced by the other cases I had to treat. I also shared my results and recipes so that as many people as possible could benefit from the advantages of traditional Chinese medicine.

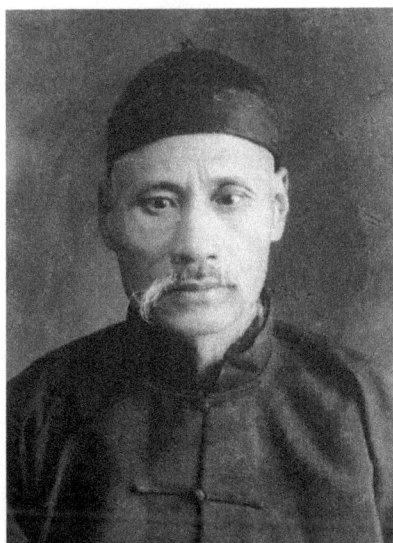

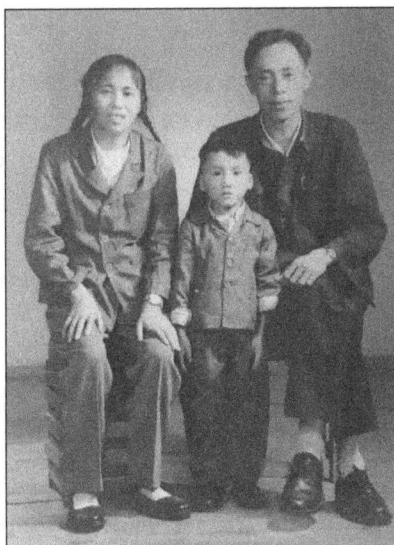

My great-grandfather, Zhiping
Dai, also a traditional doctor
and regional mayor (乡长)

My grandmother, Zhefei
Dai and my grandfather,
Baochi Cai, with my father.

The Eight Principles of Diagnosis (八纲辨证)

We are talking about Covid-19, but for us, as traditional Chinese doctors, every case is different. For example, in a family that is a victim of the pandemic, even when the source of the virus is the same, it is likely that the symptoms will differ according to age, gender, body energy, etc. Consequently, traditional Chinese medicine will adapt the treatment options to each individual.

To this end, our ancestors developed a system called the "Eight Principles of Diagnosis," based on the eight origins of symptoms which they identified as follows:

– 阴: yin;
– 阳: yang;

– 表: biǎo : superficial (yang), (localization, rather rapid, acute);
– 里: lǐ : internal (yin), (Localization, rather slow, chronic);
– 热: rè: heat (yang), (Nature, rather fast, acute);
– 寒: hán: cold (yin), (Nature, rather slow, chronic);
– 实: shí: excess (yang), (Nature, rather fast, acute);
– 虚: xū : deficiency (yin), (Nature, rather slow, chronic).

One single disease can correspond to several of these symptom origins. There are four important steps to determine them: inspection, listening, investigation, and pulse measurement. In a period of confinement, pulse measurement and inspection are impossible, which leaves listening and investigation, including tongue analysis. Here is the questionnaire that I developed specifically for Covid-19, taking into account these exceptional remote circumstances:

In this period of the Covid-19 epidemic, according to the information communicated by the health establishments in France, if you suffer from one of these three main symptoms, it is possible that you are infected:
1. 失去嗅觉 / Loss of sense of smell and taste;
2. 高烧不退 / High and persistent fever;
3. 腹泻 / Diarrhea.

In this case, please answer the following questions:

1. Express the symptoms of your illness as accurately and in as much detail as possible.
2. Have you been coughing?
3. If so, with mucus?
4. If yes, what color is it: white or yellow?

5. The color and appearance of your cheek (in the majority of cases, white cheeks indicate a Yin disease, while red cheeks indicate a Yang disease).

6. The color of your lips: pale, bright red, dark red, dry?

7. Frequency and detail of urine and stool?

8. Detail for the three meals of your daily eating habits?

9. Sleep status?

10. Are your hands and feet cold or warm?

11. With perspiration? When? Which part(s) of the body? Intensity?

12. Are you taking antibiotics or medication? If yes, which ones?

13. Inhale deeply through your mouth and then expel through your nose, tell me what you feel afterwards.

14. Send me two pictures of your tongue taken in the morning, one before brushing your teeth, the other after (before, it shows the energy of the spleen and stomach, and the state of digestion; after, it shows the symptoms).

Several questions may seem surprising, but, for example, if the hands or feet are cold, it means that the blood circulation does not reach the ends of the limbs, which indicates a weakness in the body's energy, and directs the treatment to be applied.

Organ Colour Matching

One of the principles of Traditional Chinese Medicine is to match five organs to five colors, according to the table below:

Organs	Colors
Liver	Green
Heart	Red
Spleen	Brown
Lungs	White
Kidneys	Black

One of the consequences is that, if one of these organs is weak, foods that match its color should be preferred, for example, black sesame for the kidneys or red apples for the heart. As for the lungs, their color is white, so white sesame seeds will help us to find the energy to reinvigorate them.[14]

14. This section is extensively developed in *Health through Traditional Chinese Medicine*, Angelina Jingrui Cai, ed. Louise Courteau Inc. 2020.

Chapter III

Lungs and (Corona) Viruses

Introduction
Covid-19 does not only affect the lungs: all organs are affected to varying degrees, which is why symptoms as varied as insomnia, diarrhea, loss of appetite, loss of taste, etc., occur. Consequently, our philosophy is to treat the whole, for example, the heart and kidneys to sleep well, and thus boost the immune system, the spleen and the stomach to regain appetite, which allows recovering energy through food, the intestines to stop the leakage of energy due to diarrhea.

Nevertheless, the lungs play a central role in such a pandemic, so their treatment is essential.

Lungs Are Life!
According to the observations of traditional Chinese medicine, they are a Yin organ, to which the large intestine is the Yang counterpart. Indeed, this is a concept that is not easy to transcribe into English, but basically, it is considered that the organs function in Yin-Yang pairs.

Of course, they are all essential, but the lungs are critical in more ways than one:

– they control all the meridians (we'll come back to this in the next chapter);

– they are the masters of Qi, that is, of the vital energy, because they govern it, as well as breathing.

They are delicate organs, the most sensitive and fragile among all the others: they need protection and require more attention and care. Being connected with the throat and opened through the nose, they are the first organs to be contaminated in case of a virus-like Covid-19.

Properties and relations with other organs
Some symptoms of Covid-19, which do not appear to be related to the lungs, nevertheless originate from them, given the links with other organs.

1) The heart
The lungs are considered the "king's parasol" because they protect the closest organ, the heart. They help it in its circulatory function, providing it with Qi to ensure blood circulation. In case of weakness, it is the whole functioning of the organs and of the body that is affected.

The consequences of Covid-19
According to traditional Chinese medicine, it is mainly the heart that dominates sleep. This explains why the majority of people affected by Covid-19 become insomniacs, even if they have little anxiety or coughing discomfort. Indeed, when the lung's energy is weakened, it is no longer able to help move energy from the heart to the kidneys, so we can no longer relax and reach the state that allows us to fall asleep. In addition, the heart continues to function like an engine running in a vacuum, with the risk of a heart attack, among other things.

2) The spleen
The lungs also protect the spleen. They transform and help to fortify the energy it produces, which is essential for blood circulation. As a result, if the energy coming from the lungs weaken, so does that

of the spleen and the efficiency of its functions decreases: it can no longer get rid of the excess water in the body, which causes water retention, edemas, nor can it stimulate the appetite, accompany the work of the stomach, etc.

The consequences of Covid-19
The links between the lungs and the spleen naturally explain symptoms such as loss of appetite, swelling of the stomach, diarrhea. Indeed, it is the spleen that dominates the appetite and manages digestion with its partner, the stomach.

3) The kidneys
Kidney function depends on the energy in the lungs. If they are sick, one of the renal consequences is the bad allocation and evacuation of water in the body, the amplification of respiratory problems, etc.

The consequences of Covid-19
Sleep is not only dominated by the heart, but the kidneys also contribute to it: to sleep well, the Yang energy of the heart must descend into the Yin energy of the kidneys.
This is why when we treat Covid-19, it is indispensable to activate the energy of the kidneys, in order to improve circulation and sleep, two fundamentals to strengthen the immune system and defeat the disease.

Covid-19 Principles and Keys

Example of diseases determination
In TCM, it is necessary to identify the origin of a disease, because even if it is a cold, it will not be treated in the same way by being of Yin or Yang origin. Here are four examples, which apply to symptoms of cold, flu and Covid-19.

– Yin
风寒 (Fēng Hán) Cold wind, or 伤寒 (Shāng Hán) Typhoid Fever / Cold Stroke.
An indication of one of these two Yin cases is the white or thick white tongue.

– Yang
风热 (Fēng Rè) Hot wind / Warm wind, or 风燥 (Fēng Zào) Dry wind.
An indication of one of these two Yang cases is a tongue that is dry, red, yellow or thick yellow.

Since Covid-19 is not identified as such in traditional Chinese medicine, here are the categories to which it is related in the classification of our ancestors:
温病 (Wēn Bîng), Warm disease
湿温 (Shī Wen), Wet and Warm Disease
疫病 (Yî Bîng) /疫疠(Yî Lî), Epidemic disease
温疫 (Wēn Yî), Warm epidemic disease
疟疾 (Nüè Ji), Malaria
痰饮 (Tán Yīn), Mucositis

邪 (or 邪气) Xie (or Xie Qi), Negative Energy
伏邪气 (or 伏气) Fú Xié Qî (or Fú Qî), Latent Negative Energy
虚 (Xu), Disability (or Void).

As a result, even if it is a single virus, Covid-19 can have a cold or hot reaction on a sick person, such as the flu or a cold, which changes its symptoms and therefore the treatments.

Prevention Advice

In a saucepan, boil three liters, five parts water and one part vinegar, and add three tablespoons of salt. After bringing it to a boil, diffuse it in all the rooms of your home.

Fengshui masters in China have been using this method for centuries, to remove harmful waves. They choose black rice vinegar, which can be bought in Asian supermarkets, as its disinfectant and antimicrobial effect is superior to that of others.

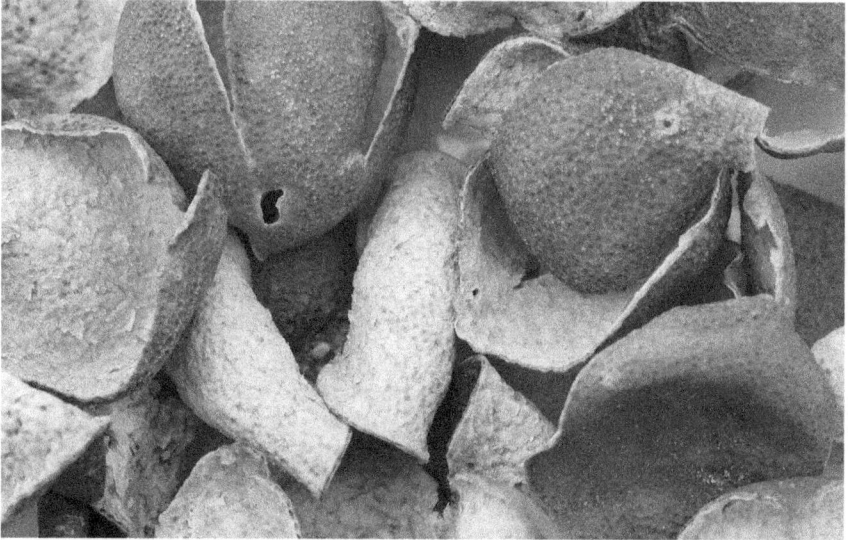

Chenpi is dried mandarin peel, which has undergone a unique drying process over several years.

Chapter IV

Meridians and Acupuncture Points

They are a key concept in traditional Chinese medicine. Meridians are invisible "channels" through which vital energy flows. There are twelve main ones. Any blockage at one point leads to disturbances that can cause illness.

A traditional doctor will then use, among other means, acupuncture points located all over the body, especially along the meridians. Nearly two thousand have been identified, but between three hundred and four hundred are used to treat most situations. In fact, part of my research involves the discovery of new acupuncture points, which could prove indispensable in treating new diseases and in coping with the evolution of the environment in general and of human beings in particular—indeed, the energy in which we bathe is no longer the same as it was even a century ago.

The concept of meridians and acupuncture points is foreign to Western science, but we use them for several techniques, some of which have proven to be valuable against Covid-19.

1. Moxibustion

Feeling of Warmth

According to traditional Chinese medicine, this very ancient method ranks among the best, if not the best, for preventing and treating diseases. In fact, the TCM bible says to use it if you can't cure with herbs or acupuncture. Moreover, as many plants can produce side effects, it is recommended to apply moxibustion afterwards, in order to repair the affected organs, as well as after the use of suction cups, to recharge the energy.

It is also a significant accompaniment to acupuncture, which Chinese name 针灸 (Zhen (Jiu), is composed of 针 (Zhen), which means "acupuncture," and 灸 (Jiu) which means "moxibustion."

To obtain a more effective result in acupuncture, TCM, therefore, recommends that it be accompanied by moxibustion.

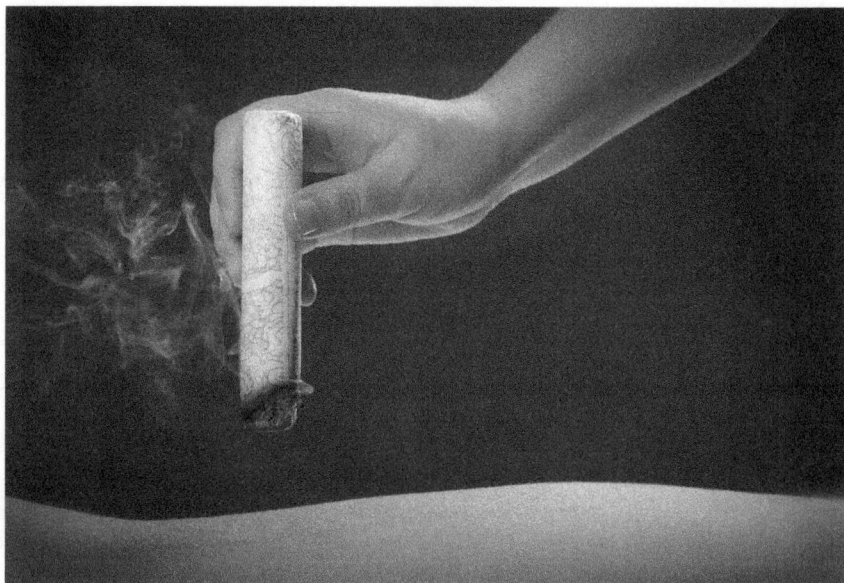

Sagebrush Practice

Moxibustion is a relatively simple technique: it includes heating points of the body with a moxa, that is to say, a stick made of mugwort leaves that you burn. It is considered that the mugwort cotton, producing the most Yang energy, i.e. the most efficient ones, come from the Chinese province of Hubei, of which the capital is Wuhan.

The force of the moxa's Yang energy can penetrate the meridians and even the viscera.

There are moxibustion boxes, which facilitate the practice. In this case, a "cube" (in fact a 3 cm long cylinder) is used, while the stick is about 20 cm long (see photos). If you do not have a specific box, do not bring the stick closer than 4 cm to the skin, which is about twice the diameter of the moxa.

The moxibustion time for each acupuncture point is about twenty minutes, i.e. the time it takes for a (small) moxa to burn out (the stick can be used up to five times, as it lasts longer).

In a normal period, i.e. in good health, it is sufficient to practice moxibustion for three days to strengthen our energy.

When you practice on at least two points consecutively, it is necessary to follow the general order recommended by traditional Chinese medicine: starting from the upper points and progressing towards the lower ones, and from left to right, because it is always necessary to start from the Yang side (top/left) to the Yin side (bottom/right), in order to follow the direction of the energy flow. The opposite can cause disorder and dysfunction, including nervousness. If you have acquired a moxibustion device with three boxes, you can treat three points at the same time. Otherwise, follow the order indicated.

There is no need to wait or pause between points.

Drink lukewarm water before moxibustion to facilitate the release of blockages in the energy circulation and increase its efficiency, as well as afterwards to help evacuate blockages (humidity, waste, cold).

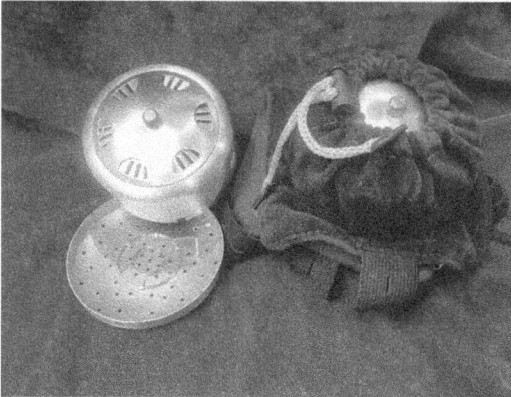

Moxibustion box...

...and with a moxa starting to burn off before the box is closed

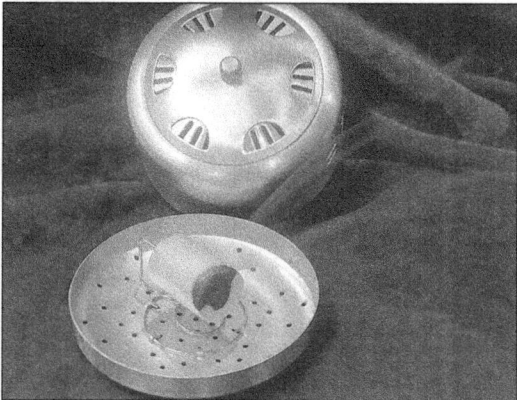

Contraindications

As moxibustion generates an excess of blood circulation, it is not recommended:
- for pregnant women;
- during the menstrual period if menstruation is heavy;
- for people suffering from high blood pressure.

Given its benefits, it may nevertheless be useful to seek the advice of a professional of traditional Chinese medicine.

It is also not advisable to practice it while eating, after eating too much, when you are hungry or drink too much alcohol because the circulation of energy is then disrupted, which reduces its effectiveness.

Properties

Among its main effects, traditional Chinese medicine has established that moxibustion enhances vitality, chases away cold, dehumidifies the body, promotes blood circulation and, in general, improves the immune system's resistance by balancing the Yin and Yang energies.

Moxa has antibacterial and antiviral effects and using as well as smoke from its leaves in specific circumstances can inhibit the action of certain viruses, including the flu.

In this period of Covid-19, it is even recommended to burn it at home or at work, like incense, to purify the air and reduce the risk of contamination.

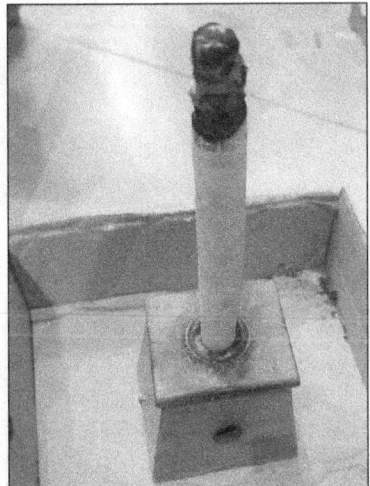

Moxa stick burning in a shop

Three Key Points

Of the hundreds of points on which moxibustion can be performed, at least three are particularly effective against Covid-19, and any lung infection in general. Unlike other techniques, such as acupuncture, it is not necessary to locate the point with extreme precision, as the effect occurs on the area. That said, it is still better not to be too far away from the points.

It should be noted that it is not always easy to locate the points, especially when you are beginning, but it comes with practice.

1) Da Zhui (大椎), DU14

Location: it is an energy collection point located on the spine, at the bottom of the seventh cervical vertebra. To find it, raise your head high: it is located in the hollow of the neck, above the shoulder line.

Indications: fever, cough, cold, bronchitis, redness of the skin, swelling of the belly, night sweats, eye pain, stiffness of the neck, asthma, epilepsy.

This is one of the most critical points for "freeing the outside" and treating "the heat of the wind," which generates the illnesses related to cold and heat.

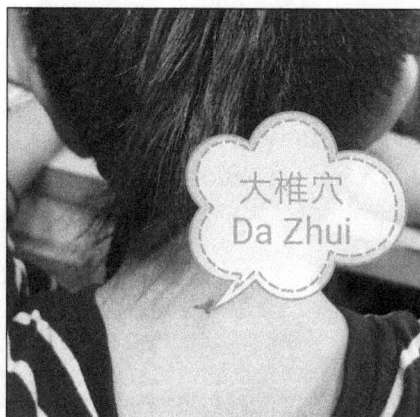

大椎穴
Da Zhui

2) Fei Shu (肺俞), BL13

Even if they are two points, they have the same name and the same international reference.[15]

Location: on the back. Starting from the first vertebra in the back (the largest, at the bottom of the neck), go down to the bottom of the hollow of the third, then move 1.5 cun to the left and right of the spine.

Indications: cough, asthma, spitting blood, hot flashes, night sweats, stuffy nose.

Acting on the Fei Shu points allows, in particular, to reinforce the energy of the lungs, by balancing Yin and Yang, which is essential in the period of coronavirus.

It is not necessary to practice systematically on both points, only one can suffice, except in serious situations. If both have to be done, start with the one on the left.

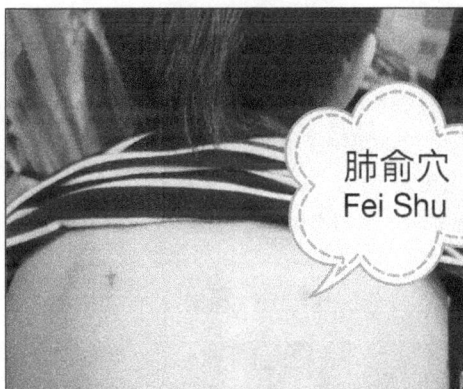

肺俞穴
Fei Shu

---

15. Professionals consider, in practice, that it is only one point, but we use this notion of "two" points in the book in order to make it easier to understand. This is also why there is only one international reference for Fei Shu and Ding Chuan

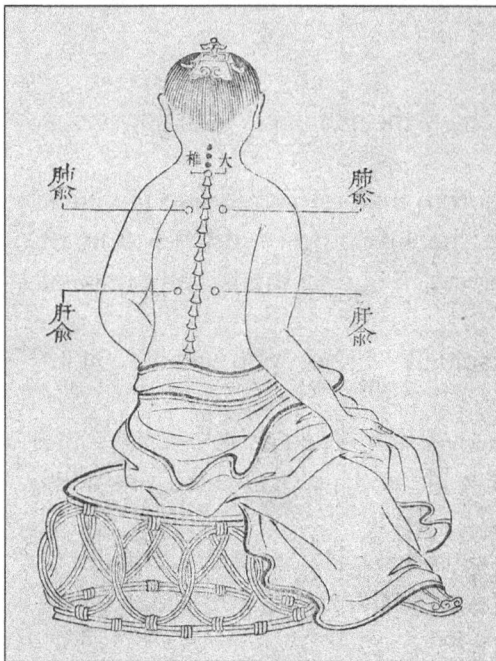

Image from an ancient medical treatise from 1680 (Qing Dynasty) showing Da Zhui, Fei Shu and Gan Shu points (for the liver).
Source: Wellcome Images / Wikimedia Commons

3) Ding Chuan (定喘), EX-B1

"定喘" means "stopping the breathing block." These are two specific points that are not in the twelve main meridians.

Location: they are located on the back. Starting from the first vertebra in the back (the largest), go down to the bottom of the hollow of the seventh and then deviate 0.5 cun to the left and right of the spine.

Indications: asthma, cough, stiff neck, shoulder and back pain.

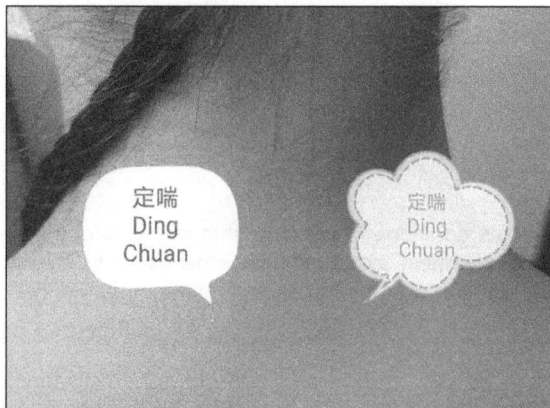

A Personal Measure: the Cun (寸)

In traditional Chinese medicine the "cun," a unit of measurement for locating acupuncture points, is often used. It is based on the principle of dividing the body into equal segments, the number of which is the same regardless of a person's size. Thus, a baby and an adult will have precisely the same number of cuns on all parts of the body: they will have, for example, the same number of cuns on the leg.

As a result, the cun is not a universal fixed value, as the meter can be: each person has his or her own cun, which depends on the width of the thumb and fingers, the real determiners of each person's cun.

This way, we can approximately locate the area where our acupuncture points are located, the exact position being felt by touch.

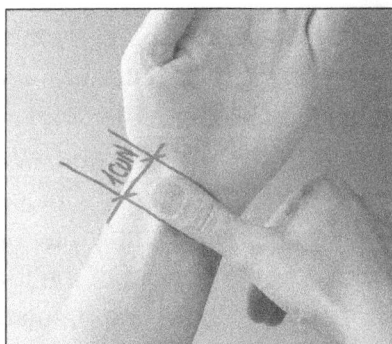

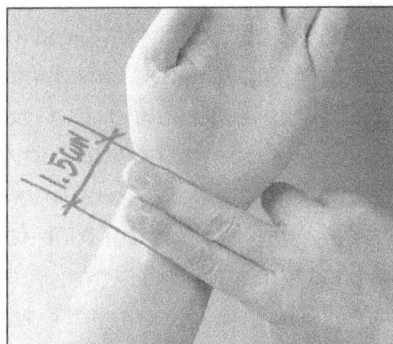

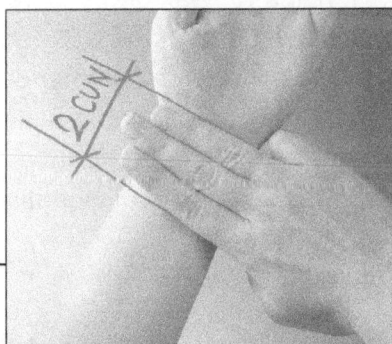

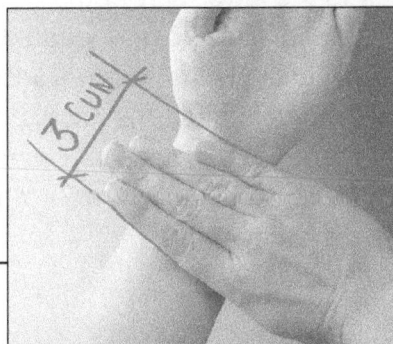

Instructions for Use

I often advise to moxibustion Da Zhui then Fei Shu points, except in case of difficulty breathing, where it is more efficient to use the combination Da Zhui then Ding Chuan—follow the order recommended by traditional Chinese medicine, as explained above. As a reminder, you should therefore start with Da Zhui, then Fei Shu on the left, followed by Fei Shu on the right, and not the other way around.

The practice of moxibustion does not present any danger or side effect - there may however be a form of apprehension, at least the first time, for fear of burning oneself. Granted, but in more than two decades of practice, none of my patients has ever burned themselves or asked me to relieve a burn due to moxibustion.

I recommend moxibustion sessions preferably in the morning for the points located at the top of the chest, therefore those related to Yang energy; otherwise in the evening the risk is to energize it, thus generating insomnia.

However, especially in most cases of Covid-19, the symptoms of (violent) coughing and difficulty breathing also interfere with sleep, while exhausting the body and weakening the immune system. So do not hesitate to practice in the evening and even at night if necessary. Even more so because traditional Chinese medicine has known the trick for a long time: you simply have to add a moxibustion point which is located at the bottom of the foot and called Yong Quan (涌泉), which means "to bring Yang energy back to the lower part of the body." It helps to relax and ensure a good sleep—this point is located at the lower part of the body and should conclude the session, according to the order recommended by TCM. As is often the case, one point may be enough, so start with the left foot in case you would need to do the other foot.

This also works if you are not sick... So if you're an insomniac, here's a hint for you!

Results

Of the hundred or so people who approached me, I recommended moxibustion to almost all of them. However, due to the lack of moxa available during the confinement period, only about 40% were able to apply the advice. According to their feedback, the results are satisfactory, and there have been no relapses. In fact, I have recommended that moxibustion be continued after healing, to continue to strengthen the inner energy and repair the organs affected by Covid-19, using Da Zhui and then Fei Shu first.

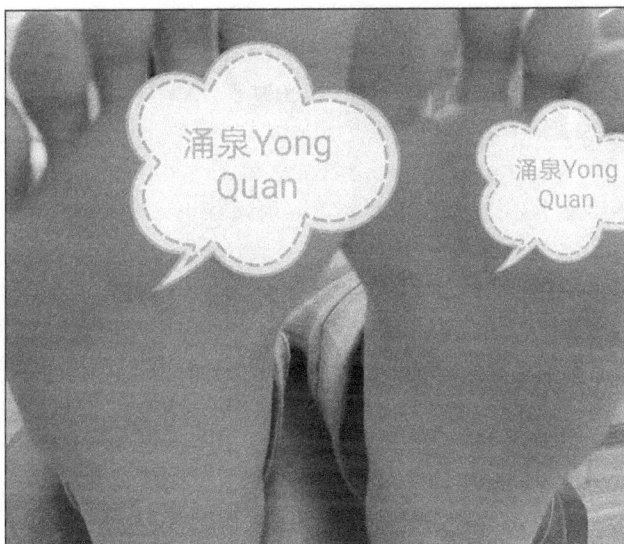

2. The Suction Pads

Millennia Old, but Still Modern

It is an ancient technique, which has also been known in Europe for a long time, as Hippocrates was already using it in 400 BC. It is beneficial to treat muscular, articular and rheumatic pains, and many pulmonary pathologies, including Covid-19, the flu. In fact, it was the first treatment I used for the couple from Wuhan who came to see me.

The principle lies in the improvement of blood circulation, which has the effect of removing blockages, thus relieving and healing.

If you are equipped with a suction cup device, practice on the Da Zhui and Fei Shu points, precisely as with moxibustion. Since this technique is designed to "unload" us, in order to help us get rid of the body's negativities, it may also weaken us. This is why moxibustion is recommended at the end of the session, to promote not only blood circulation but also to recover energy.

Unlike the other techniques presented in this chapter, it is preferable not to practice it alone, as it is challenging to put suction cups on your back while lying on your stomach. You can also practice sitting or lying on your side. Choose the one that is most comfortable for you.

What Material?

There are suction cups made of glass, bamboo and plastic. For personal, non-professional use, the plastic version is more suitable, because those made of glass or bamboo need to be heated first, in order to empty the air, and a small clumsy gesture can cause burns and injuries.

Plastic suction cups with a pump allow practical and quick use (see photo). They can be fixed or used as a massage tool coupled with essential oil.

Moreover, thanks to the pump gun and the hose, this model facilitates the placement on the back for points that are difficult to reach when you are alone, such as Da Zhui, Fei Shu, Ding Chuan i.e. points against Covid-19, flu, colds...

Instructions for Use

Place the suction cup on the target point, lift the upper piston of the selected tank to ensure ventilation, then pump with the gun (about ten times), until the skin swells, and leave it for about ten minutes (just lift the piston at the end of the treatment). Those suffering from airway blockages will find that the skin color in the suction cups often turns red, purple or black. Basically, the darker the color (purple or black), the more serious the disease.

These traces usually disappear quickly, but they may remain for up to a few days, depending on the person and their state of energy circulation.

Sometimes water vapor appears on the walls of the suction cups, which means that there is excess moisture in the body.

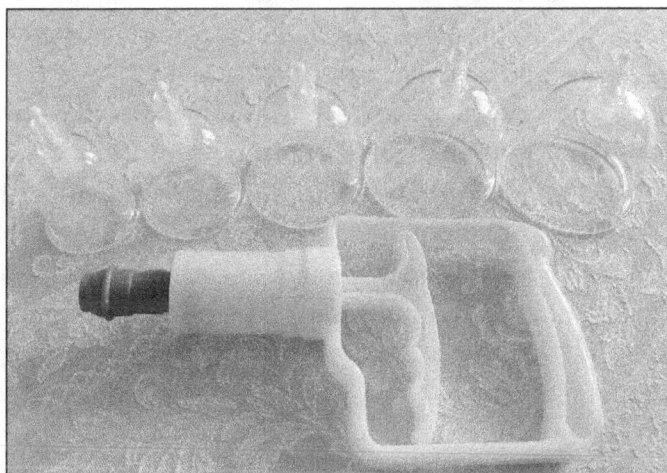

Recommendations

In normal situations, i.e. outside of a Covid-19 or flu epidemic, it is recommended to use the suction cups preferably in spring and summer, but not in autumn or winter, as this is the period of energy storage and they have the effect of discharging it.

From a hygienic point of view, it is essential to use one's suction cups and to wash and disinfect them with alcohol after each use.

Results

Especially in this period of confinement when the stores were closed, few of the people who approached me had the proper equipment. So I recommended this solution only a few times. Here is the example of Mrs. Z., who is fifty-five years old. She contacted me on April 11th with the usual symptoms of Covid-19: greasy cough, difficulty breathing, insomnia, fever, loss of smell and taste. She had been following her doctor's prescription for two weeks, without any improvement, which worried her more and more.

Her tongue was white and thick, with a yellow layer. Considering the other symptoms, my recommendations were similar to several cases presented in the previous pages: my grandmother's recipe to remove fever (garlic + ginger + chives), foot baths with about ten slices of ginger + 50 g of mulberry leaves for insomnia, morning and evening infusion for seven days of 50 g of Chenpi + 20 g of liquorice + Yu Ping Feng San + 50 g of Artemisia. And as she was equipped with suction cups, I recommended her to practice twice a week on the now well-known points of Dazhui, Feishu and Ding Chuan, to be completed afterwards by a moxibustion session.

A week later, she was breathing normally again, the cough had almost disappeared, and she had regained her sense of taste and smell. She was completely cured ten days after my recommendations, that is to say within three sessions of suction cups. Of course, it is impossible to attribute this success to the suction cups alone, since she followed the whole program, but she then recommended this system to her entourage in France and China. She told me that several of her friends had found it to be effective in calming coughs and returning to fluid breathing.

Let's add two examples to illustrate the use of suction cups with other health issues:

1) Mr. L.'s parents had been coughing for a month with no solution. I suggested that they used suction cups, information that he passed on to his parents in China. Later, he confirmed that two sessions were enough to cure them.

2) Mr. Y. lives in Val-de-Marne (Paris Region). Allergic to pollen, he couldn't breathe properly. He regained normal breathing after four sessions of suction cups, each time accompanied by moxibustion. Indeed, as indicated above, even if spring and summer are the right seasons to use the suction cups to get rid of blockages, finishing off with moxibustion remains essential, in order to boost our energy.

3. The Needles

In case of sore throat, cough, nervousness, we can use a traditional Chinese method, with a pin or a needle. It is all the more effective as it is used early, as soon as the symptoms appear.

Start by burning the tip with a lighter or a match to disinfect it. Then, it is essential to rub the area thoroughly before inserting the needle to ensure a better release of the blockage. This will also reduce the stinging sensation.

Next, make the indicated point(s) lightly bleed until the color of the blood changes from dark to normal, i.e. bright red. A sore throat means that part of the lungs is inflamed. Automatically, the blood color becomes darker, especially on these points.

After the bleeding, disinfect the skin with a little alcohol and apply cotton wool for a few seconds.

Typically, the symptoms will disappear in a single session. If this is not enough, wait at least until the next day to start again.

In the case of Covid-19, two points can be particularly useful. These are by the way the ones I have recommended to the people who have solicited me.

1) Shào Shāng (少商), LU11
Logically, it has an impact on lung disease, as it is the eleventh point on the lung meridian.
It is 0.1 cun outside the bottom of the left or right thumbnail.
Its properties: soothes coughs, removes throat pain, reduces fever, is effective for colds, angina or pneumonia, also used for mental disorders.

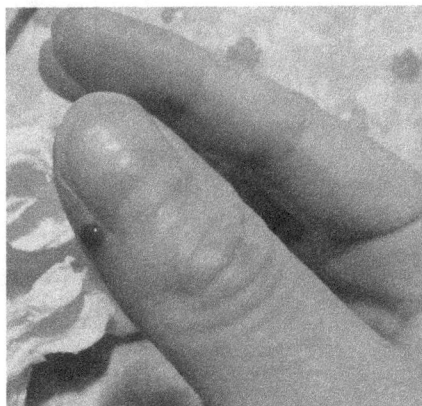

Shào Shāng (少商), LU11   Shāng Yáng (商阳), LI1

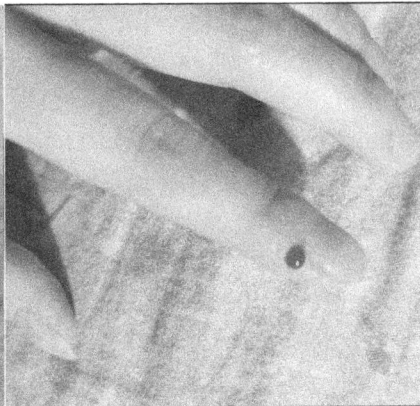

2) Shāng Yáng (商阳), LI1

It is the first point on the meridian of the large intestine, which is the Yang "partner" of the Yin lungs. It may seem surprising to have to act on the gut meridian in the case of Covid-19. In fact, TCM explains that one of the functions of the lungs is to bring down Qi energy so that, among other things, the large intestine can work properly, i.e. that its motility[16] and digestion are optimal. If they are blocked, the intestinal meridian will not function properly, causing symptoms such as diarrhea or constipation. Reciprocally, if the intestinal meridian is not at its best, then the meridian in the lungs will not function properly either, which will lead to sore throats, coughing, etc.

This point is 0.1 cun outside the bottom of the left or right index nail.

Its properties: it removes nervousness, helps to regulate digestion, relieves throat or dental pain, reduces swelling in the stomach.

---

16. Motility is "the ability of an organism to move independently, using metabolic energy." Source: Wikipedia.

Shào Shāng (少商) and Shāng Yáng (商阳) are two of the "Jing" (井) or "well" points. They are often used in cases of fainting and unconsciousness, for example, after a stroke. In this case, the patient should be treated as soon as possible. If disinfected needles are not available, press hard with your fingernails and hold for at least two minutes on each point, starting with Shāng Yáng (商阳), then Shào Shāng (少商).

This is a technique I had used on many occasions, including twice on an airplane, when the flight attendants called for emergency medical attention after a hypoglycemic attack in a passenger who had lost consciousness, as well as a case where a violent asthma attack was threatening to suffocate a young woman.

Results

Out of the hundred or so people I was consulted, only about ten of them opted for this method, according to the feedback I received — it may take courage to prick yourself and bleed, but sometimes in life, misfortunes go away through the pain. So for these ten people, the results were spectacular, with almost immediate relief and symptoms are gone the next day.

Here are two cases:

1) A person in Italy, cousin of a French friend, open to traditional Chinese medicine. Towards the end of March, she tested positive, with rather important symptoms such as fever up to 38,5 °C, violent cough outbreaks, loss of appetite, loss of taste and smell, digestive disorders, diarrhea, difficulties breathing.

The color of her tongue was a thick white, which reflects a worrying state of health — I could hardly understand what she was explaining to me, as her words were regularly interspersed with coughing fits. Therefore, I recommended that she used the needles immediately, in order to soothe this horrible cough, and then tried the following recipes:

– my grandmother's recipe for removing fever (garlic + ginger + chives);

– an infusion of Chinese absinthe (50 g) + Yu Ping Feng San + 50 g of Chenpi + 10 g of liquorice, during one week morning and evening;

– moxibustion on the three points Da Zhui, Fei Shu and Ding Chuan at least once a day;

– foot baths with ginger and mulberry leaves.

Her health improved significantly at the end of the first week, and I recommended strengthening it with Yu Ping Feng San for seven days, continuing the foot baths.

She told me that she was healed entirely two weeks after our first contact.

2) A French-Chinese family called me for help at the beginning of the lockdown, because the husband started to present the symptoms of Covid-19: loss of appetite, sore throat, fever up to 38,5 °C. They were worried because the co-worker he shared the office with had just been diagnosed positive. The wife called the Paramedics and his GP, who advised him to stay at home and take Paracetamol. Three days later, the situation did not improve: the fever came and went, but the sore throat had intensified. Increasingly worried, they did various researches to find a solution and contacted me through WeChat.

To reduce fever, I advised drinking my grandmother's now-famous recipe. For the sore throat, I recommended the needle technique, to be practiced once every two days (no more than seven times over two weeks), until the blood color returned to 100% bright red at the beginning of the bleeding.

This family was faced with a situation that had occurred several times during lockout, namely the unavailability of the recommended plants and ingredients. So I asked them to make a list of what they could get. From that, I recommend an infusion of mint and honey to clear the respiratory tract, and also to sunbathe to replace moxibustion, ideally in the late morning (except in summer, when it is better to expose oneself earlier).

A week later, the wife confirmed to me that the fever was gone since the first pricking, that the sore throat had also disappeared and that her husband was beginning to regain his appetite. Since then, everything has been fine.

If needles do not tempt you, there are other possibilities, including Gua Sha.

4. The Gua Sha (刮痧)

"Scratching Away the Disease"

It is probably one of the least renowned methods of traditional Chinese medicine in the West. Yet it is a family method, effective and ancient. Moreover, we are ending this chapter with one of the techniques recommended as first aid by TCM. Indeed, drugs, including plants, can present the risk of side effects. Therefore, if one has a choice, it is best to start with Gua Sha and/or suction cups.

The meaning of the original expression means "to scratch." This method consists in using a tool, a wooden comb or, a hand in a cat claw position, to scratch or comb the skin or back in the direction of the energy in order to "make the disease go away." The side effects are relatively small, or even non-existent, as long as you do not scratch more than is reasonable. Nevertheless, as with any technique of Traditional Chinese Medicine, it is necessary to be helped or treated by professionals in this field.

Gua Sha is mainly used to regulate Qi, promote blood circulation, reduce excess Yang energy in the lungs, relax muscles, soothe pain and detoxify the body by facilitating circulation and water drainage. It is also widely used in the field of beauty, as well as for the treatment of certain painful diseases, such as osteoarthritis, herniated discs, etc.

Gua Sha has also been found to facilitate rehabilitation for patients with hemiplegia following a stroke.

And one of the reasons why this technique is included in this chapter is that it can give excellent results for colds, fever, coughs, breathing difficulties, asthma, etc., which are some of the symptoms of Covid-19.

"Water From Within"

To get rid of blockages and diseases related to the lungs and airways, we look for the meridian of the lungs on the left, where there is a very important acupuncture point called Chi Ze (尺泽), which means "water from within."

Location: In a sitting position, with the palm facing upwards and the elbow slightly bent, this acupuncture point is located on the ulnar surface of the fold, outside the tendon.

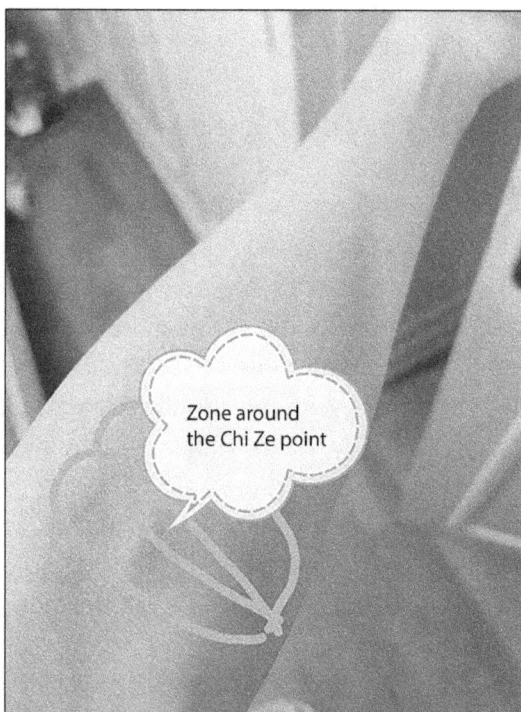

Zone around the Chi Ze point

The effectiveness of Chi Ze is due to the fact that it is the place where the Qi of the meridian accumulates and penetrates deep into the body. This point is known to strengthen the Qi energy by acting on the water in the body.

For this method, we use a wooden comb, on the handle's side, to detoxify and get rid of the mucus. First of all, we start by tapping the Chi Ze point, without worrying about precision, because it is the whole area around it that is important.

When it becomes slightly red, we take the comb and scrape from top to bottom (this is what we mean by "cleaning," to remove and drain), until red, purple, or sometimes even black spots appear.

If you feel relieved, stop, then drink a glass of lukewarm water in order to reinforce the evacuation and detoxification. Otherwise, you can practice on the other arm, in the same way. Indeed, it is not necessary to scratch both points if the problem is resolved on the first attempt.

Repeat once every two days if the problem recurs, for a week.

Before rubbing, apply a thin layer of coconut or olive oil, which are more natural than the so-called "massage" oils, as their composition is not always known, and some ingredients may cause side effects.

Warning: people who suffer from blood problems or diabetes should not try Gua Sha, at least not without a doctor's advice.

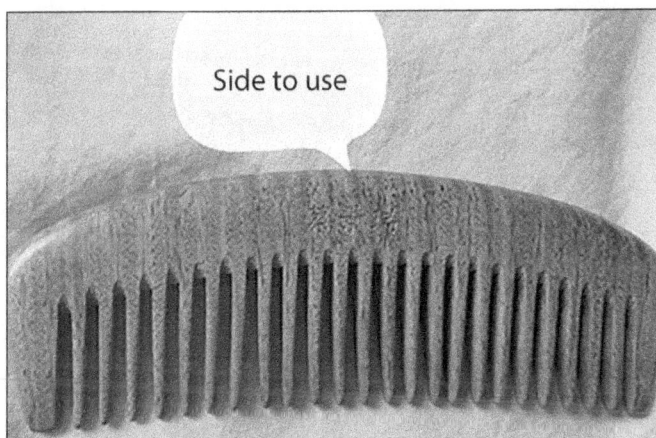

Side to use

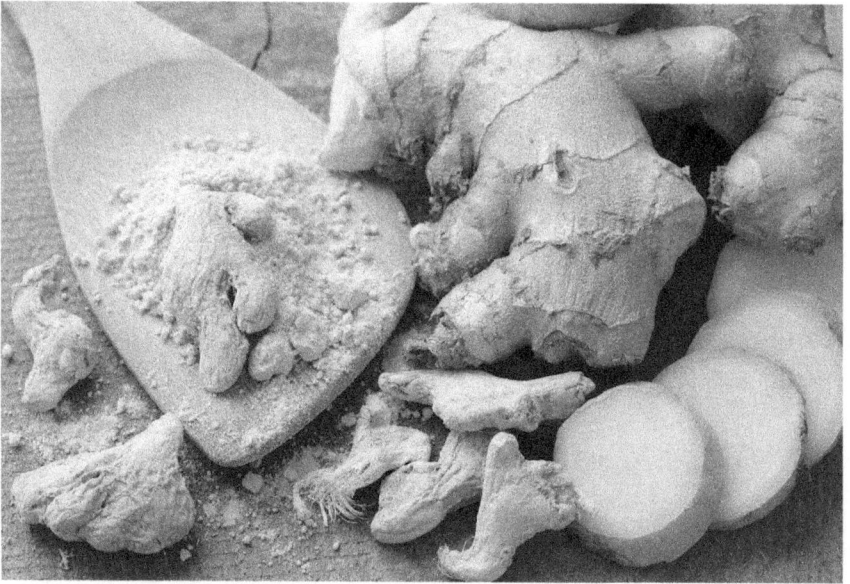

Ginger

Chapter V

Nutrition, Recipes and Techniques
Against Covid-19 and Other Viruses

Nutrition is a crucial element of traditional Chinese medicine, according to the principle well known in the West: "May your food be your medicine."

All the products listed in the recipes below can be purchased in Asian and specialty supermarkets, and increasingly in other stores.

Some of these recipes do not have a direct effect on the symptoms of Covid-19, but they do help to strengthen the immune system and are therefore essential for boosting natural defenses and prevention.

1. A Soup From my Grandmother

According to traditional Chinese medicine, if the body temperature is below 37 °C, it indicates a lack of energy. However, it has been observed for some years now, because the urban lifestyle takes us away from nature and its Yang energy, and due to a lack of exercise, that we are no longer always able to maintain the body at this temperature, which causes a lack of Yang energy.

On the other hand, if the temperature rises, fever is the sign that the immune system is fighting germs. As of 39 °C, it is too weakened, and we must then use other solutions than those presented in this book.

It so happens that the many cases (of symptoms) of Covid-19 that I have been confronted with almost all had a fever, but rarely above 38 °C or even 38.5 °C maximum. This is the limit at which this recipe is effective.

Here it is: in a saucepan, boil the equivalent of a large bowl of water, with three heads of grated garlic, five slices of ginger and three branches of chopped Thai chives, selecting only the white parts.

As long as the temperature of the beverage does not allow you to drink it, bring it close to your face to use the steam to clear your airways.

The taste isn't great, but you must drink the entire bowl, hot and without adding other ingredients, such as sugar or even honey. Normally, you should start sweating and then watch the fever gradually disappear thanks to the sweating. Generally, it only takes one time to get rid of it. However, if it persists or comes back, you can reiterate three times, but only once a day.

During this period of Covid-19, I recommended this recipe to about 40 people with fever, including those mentioned at the beginning of the book. In the majority of cases, the fever went away in one go, at most three times in the case of a person with persistent fever with a high temperature.

2. Two Footbath Recipes

It is a little-known practice in the West, yet it is simple and effective, without danger or side effects (except for excess tension, as already mentioned above). Here are two recipes particularly indicated in cases of Covid-19, flu, colds, especially for their effect on sleep:

A) As we have seen previously, I have repeatedly recommended foot baths with about ten slices of ginger + 50 g of mulberry leaves. This composition is to be preferred to relax before going to sleep.

B) This recipe is used to remove fever and, at the same time, relax (a little less than with formula A): in three liters of water, boil 100 g of dried moxa leaves + 100 g of dried safflower flowers. Pour into a container, adding cold or lukewarm water to bring the water temperature down to about 50 °C. Dip the feet; the water should cover the ankles. Maintain the temperature for twenty to thirty minutes, adding hot water from time to time, until you start to sweat slightly. Practice this in the evening before going to sleep.

In the time that I have been recommending this composition, hundreds of people have successfully adopted it, including in cases of Covid-19 symptoms.

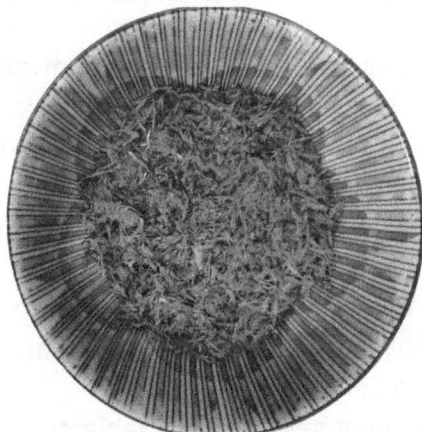

Dried Safflowers

3. *The Houttuynia Cordata* (鱼腥草)

In the Chinese pharmacopoeia, there is a plant that is very effective in fighting infections of the pulmonary and urinary tracts and, in general, all infections related to humidity. Its Latin name is *Houttuynia cordata* (鱼腥草).

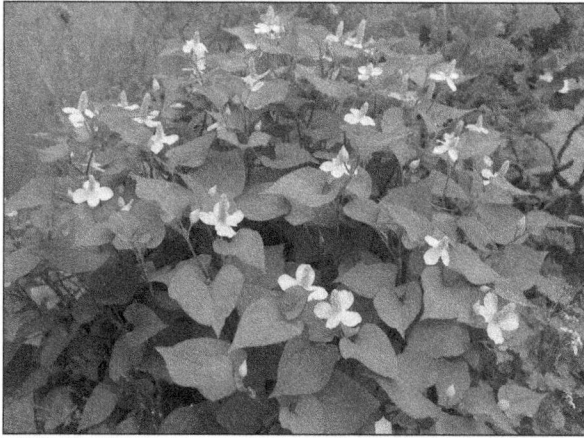

Among its many properties, the most important in times of Covid-19 and flu are: improves lung inflammation; unblocks and purifies the respiratory tract. As it is a Yin plant, its consumption must be moderate; otherwise, it will generate a Yang deficiency in the long run.

You can prepare it as a salad:

– wash and cut 150 g of branches and leaves, mix with a head of grated garlic (of a slightly warm nature), which allows obtaining the balance between Yin and Yang energies;

– add a tablespoon of sesame oil, a tablespoon of soy sauce, a little lemon juice or chilli sauce.

A piece of advice for lovers: as the taste is strong, it is best to eat this dish together, so that you can both smell of garlic!

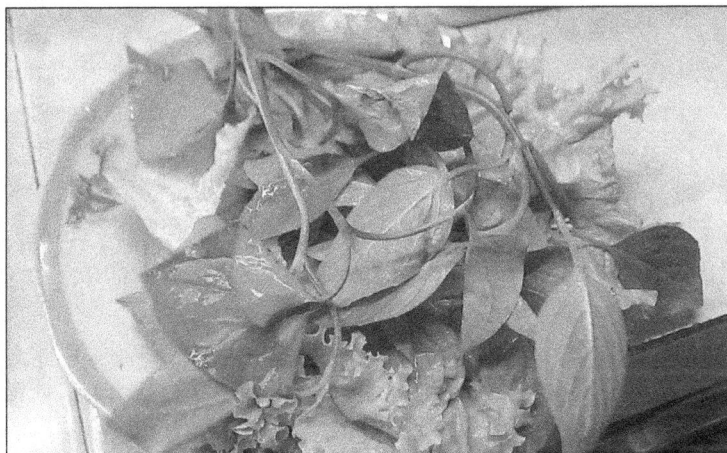

About twenty people followed my recommendations and tested this salad for their sore throats: in most cases, they only needed to eat it for lunch for three days to get the desired results. It's best to avoid eating it in the evening, because being of a Yin nature, it can weaken the stomach and generate gastric reflux, which will disturb sleep.

It can also be used as an infusion: 10 to 20 g of dried leaves in a cup are enough. It is an infusion to be avoided in the evening before going to sleep.

4. Lemongrass

It is a miraculous plant, known especially in Europe for its anti-mosquito properties, in the form of candles, incense or essential oils. Very present in Thai cuisine, it is also a true medicinal plant, to be used in decoction and infusion for internal use, or as an essential oil to be applied on the skin.

As it is related to the meridians of the lung, stomach and bladder, its properties are numerous: digestive and soothing virtues, anti-inflammatory, antispasmodic, antibacterial, anti-cellulite.

It is also recognized as useful:

– against diabetes, by lowering the blood sugar level;

– for the treatment of digestive and intestinal disorders, reducing flatulence and stomach cramps (with one cup after a meal);

– in case of joint or muscle pain, including arthritis, rheumatism, sprains, tendonitis.

– against stress, anxiety, and in case of sleep disorders, thanks to its sedative action on the nervous system. One cup after the meal is often enough to have sweet dreams;

– against fever, colds, coughs, flu-like states and, of course, Covid-19 (it was, for example, recommended as an infusion to Mrs. A.). Three daily herbal teas can then help us get through these delicate periods.

The way we use lemongrass depends on the benefits we are looking for, and it certainly hasn't finished surprising us!

Lemongrass Recipe

For colds, coughs, chest and abdominal pain: take 15 to 30 g of lemongrass leaves, boil three bowls of water, then reduce over low heat to a single bowl. Take twice a day, morning and evening after meals.

I rarely recommend lemongrass powder, because it loses some of its properties. It is better to choose the leaves.

Remarks
– to prepare an infusion, infuse 15 g of fresh lemongrass leaves in 1.5 l of water. As they have filaments that can cause lesions in the digestive tract, it is essential to filter infusions and decoctions. Otherwise, they will be difficult to digest.
– contra-indication of lemongrass: do not give to children under ten years old, because they are often in Yang over-energy, nor to people deficient in Yin, because its nature is tepid (= slightly Yang), which may further reduce their Yin energy.

Results
As this infusion is lukewarm, I recommended it to people mainly with cough symptoms as well as with breathing and digestive problems namely about eighty people, with positive feedback.
In addition to Mrs. A., let us present three cases, interesting in various ways:

Case 1: A sixty-five-year-old lady with joint pain that was increasingly unbearable, both day and night, which prevented her from sleeping. She had not been able to recover with the usual treatments, and the outbreak of the pandemic added anxiety and fear to her situation.
I recommended that she infused 500 grams of lemongrass leaves and poured them into a bathtub to take a bath. Surprisingly, the

pain went away after two days of this "treatment" and she "slept like a baby," as she said. She had even seen an improvement in her diabetes problem. She found this result so miraculous that she told me she would recommend it to everyone she knows.

Case 2: Mr. Z., fifty-one years old, was diagnosed with Covid-19. He wished to be hospitalized but was not accepted. As I saw that his condition was getting worse, I intervened personally with the hospital, which sent an ambulance in an emergency. I had done this type of intervention for at least a dozen people, for example, because they felt reassured to be taken care of in a health institution or because the confinement did not allow me to intervene directly with them when their condition required it. In any case, I have already indicated that western and traditional Chinese medicines are complementary.

When he returned home, he could no longer digest, his stomach was swollen, he had lost his appetite and still had mucus in his throat. I noticed that his tongue was still white and thick. I, therefore, advised him, to start with lemongrass infusions, in a proportion of about 50 g in 200 cl of water, to be taken three times a day after meals. He called me three days later: his belly was no longer swollen, he had regained his appetite, and the mucus had decreased a lot. To improve his condition, I recommended other recipes from this book, including moxibustion.

Case 3: In the middle of the pandemic, a French friend working as a volunteer to make cloth masks called me because of toe pain and swollen feet, due to the overload of work on her sewing machine, which prevented her from continuing. I recommended foot baths with 200 g of lemongrass and 100 g of ginger. She thanked me warmly afterwards, having evaluated the pain reduction to 70% from the first foot bath. She renewed the practice three times a day for two days, and the pain and swelling disappeared. Afterwards, she could resume making masks. Perhaps these extra masks, at a time when there weren't enough for everyone, and therefore the lemongrass, saved people from Covid-19?

5. The Fig

In TCM, this delicious fruit is considered to have effects on the meridians linked to the lungs, stomach and intestines. Here are its main properties: it promotes lung energy; regulates the Qi; calms coughs and reduces expectoration; eliminates nervousness; tones spleen energy; suppresses diarrhea; helps circulate intestinal energy; facilitates digestion; and breastfeeding.

It has also been found that figs can reduce fat deposits in blood vessels, which can lower blood pressure and prevent coronary heart diseases.

Here is a recipe for a soup or herbal tea for throat disorders (itching, pain or inflammation), including cough, asthma, Covid-19, flu, but also diarrhea: mix 70 g of fresh or dried figs depending on the season; pour into a large bowl of water and add a few lumps of white cane sugar (yellow tongue, dry cough) or full-bodied brown sugar (white tongue or thick layer). Boil, then drink and swallow the fruit twice a day for five to seven days until the symptoms disappear.

Results
The fig is currently an out-of-season product, but it can be eaten dried. The majority of people who have tried it in my groups have given me positive feedback. Among them, eight women and three men succeeded in suppressing their diarrhea after two days of consuming the recipe above.

One of them also told me that she was surprised to find that her blood pressure had returned to normal after three days of infusion three times a day. Similarly, Mrs. Y., seventy-five years old, had been suffering from a sore throat for several days, without finding success with the usual treatments. After three days of infusion of dried figs, she was cured.

6. The Dandelion

Have you observed that hundreds of small yellow suns illuminate the lawns? These are dandelions or lion-teeth (蒲公英) in bloom! The best time to pick them is mostly between April and May before flowering and always being careful to respect the environment and nature.

The medicinal virtues of this plant have been known for a long time, and not only in Asia. Here are the main ones, classified by organ:

– lungs: removes throat pain, nervousness and compensates for Yin deficiency;

– liver: purifies and removes fat, eliminates blockages that can cause red or swollen eyes, runny eyes.

– bladder: diuretic effect and facilitates urinary evacuation ;

– spleen: decreases water retention, oedemas.

Overall: reduces diabetes, blood pressure, cholesterol.

Contraindication

Dandelion is a Yin plant; therefore, consumption is not recommended for people with Yang deficiency, low Yang energy of the spleen, having too much acidity in the stomach... In that case do not take more than two meals a week with dandelions, and accompany them with slightly Yang plants, such as basil, coriander, arugula...

Dandelion Recipes

In a Salad
To be prepared with arugula leaves (of a slightly Yang nature and related to the lungs), for people who tend to be in low Yang energy or Yin over-energy. Respect the proportion of one part dandelion for two parts arugula.

Sauce for two people:
- two tablespoons of lemon sauce or fresh lemon juice;
- one and a half spoons of soy sauce;
- two spoonfuls of sesame oil.

Add, if possible, a handful of black and white sesame seeds (to be sautéed over low heat in a saucepan). The many properties of sesame are presented in the next chapter.

Sautés
Plunge the dandelions into a pot of boiling water with a teaspoon of salt for barely a minute to remove the sometimes bitter taste, then drain and cut them into pieces of about 5 centimeters. Heat two tablespoons of olive oil, then brown a head of grated garlic, before pouring in the dandelions and frying them. Add a little salt, and the dish is ready.

In Soup
In the case of Covid-19, consumption of dandelion soup is not recommended for patients with diarrhea.

In Ravioli
It's an original way to prepare them, which even children usually love. Here's the recipe:

Dandelion Ravioli
(personal recipe tested many times)

To prepare about 50 ravioli, buy one or two packs of gyoza leaves, as they are ready to use (you need one per ravioli). Here are the ingredients for the stuffing:

– 1 kg of pork meat (minced breast);

– 200 g of Bai Cai white Chinese cabbage (its sweet taste softens the bitter taste of dandelion);

– 400 g of dandelion leaves;

– 50 g of water chestnut (马蹄, Mǎ tí, an aquatic plant of Asian origin), for its lung-purifying properties and for softening the bitter taste of dandelions, thanks to its sweet flavor;

– 50 g of dehydrated scented mushrooms (to be soaked in warm water for thirty minutes);

– 10 g of garlic.

Chop all the ingredients and mix them well to make the stuffing. Add one tablespoon of salt, two tablespoons of oyster sauce, 1/4 teaspoon of Szechuan pepper powder.

For a better taste, add two tablespoons of sesame oil.

Put the stuffing in the ravioli leaves, then fold them in half. There is a device called "Gioza mould" to serrate the edge, which is very easy to use.

Cooking: Heat a saucepan and add two or three tablespoons of olive oil. As soon as white smoke appears, brown the ravioli on the flat side and add water up to half the height of the ravioli. Close with a lid until the water is completely absorbed, it's ready!

Serve with a mixture of soy sauce (1/2) and rice vinegar (1/2).

Results

I recommended dandelions for people with symptoms of Covid-19, especially when they had yellow tongues and sore throats. Cooked alone or with arugula or basil, the results were generally satisfactory.

For example, for Mrs. L.'s children, who were coughing and had dry throats, the situation was resolved in one day, after two salads of dandelions.

The result was the same for Mrs. U.'s children, who had similar symptoms, but the family's choice was soup, three times a day for five or six days, depending on the condition of their tongues.

A French mother, whose ten-year-old child I regularly follow, prepared dandelion ravioli for him, which he ate more willingly than if they had been cooked in a salad or soup, in order to purify his liver and thus calm his nervousness. She confirmed to me that one meal had changed the atmosphere of the house; even the father had become sweeter. It's great, isn't it?

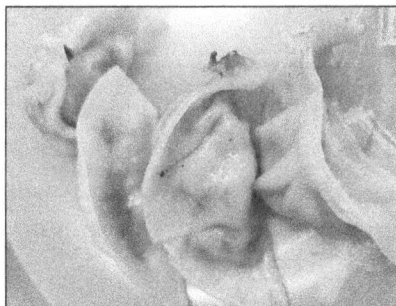

7. *Artemisia Annua* (Annual Artemisia or Chinese Wormwood—青蒿) and *Artemisia Argyi* (Chinese Artemisia—艾草)

My grandparents already used these two plants, either together or separately, especially in cases of lung infection. Taking advantage of their experience, I got into the habit of also associating them in my recommendations. When Covid-19 arrived, it was therefore quite natural that I thought they could be an adequate response, especially since they have an in depth effect on the body. So I re-studied their properties, namely according to the analyses of the book Ben Cao Gan Mu (本草纲目), and also by comparing them with various plants with similar properties. From multiple tests, I found that their results were much faster and more effective, as well as particularly adapted to the symptoms of Covid-19, such as cough, fever, diarrhea, runny nose, breathing difficulties.

In the end, I recommended this combination to more than 90% of the people who approached me, especially in critical cases, by alternating the infusion of one plant and the other, sometimes assembling them, depending on the state of health and symptoms.

Moreover, Chinese wormwood (*Artemisia annua*) is Yin. In contrast, Chinese mugwort (*Artemisia argyi*) is Yang, so the marriage of the two can neutralize the side effects coming from one energy or the other.

As a complement, I recommended most of the time foot baths every night with the recipes A) and B) presented in section 2. of this chapter, to produce the following effects: lowering fever, facilitating the circulation of Yang energy in the lungs, removing nervousness, and helping to sleep well, as many people can no longer sleep because of anxiety and stress, therefore when they are under the influence of the 恐 theme (Kǒng), "fear" in Chinese medicine.

With hindsight, the combination of these two plants seems miraculous to me, and I will continue the research because the virtues of Artemisia annua (青蒿) and Artemisia argyi (艾草) are far from having been fully discovered—they will probably enable us to treat other health problems.

An Example of Protocol

Mr. E. worked in a tobacconist's shop, where he met a lot of people every day. Five of his clients tested positive for Covid-19. In turn, the symptoms manifested themselves: thick white tongue, cough, mild fever, diarrhea, loss of appetite, sense of smell and sleep.

In the beginning, I suggested that he drank every day for a week an infusion of Chinese absinthe (50 g) + dried mandarin peel (50 g) + Yu Ping Feng San composition; practice moxibustion on Da Zhui, Fei Shu and Ding Chuan points; and take a foot bath every evening with moxa leaves and ginger.

At the end of this program, the fever disappeared, the sense of smell came back, the cough decreased, as well as the throat pain, and the sleep was soothed. His condition was much better, but he was not yet definitively cured.

As the thickness of the tongue had diminished and the color had changed, with a light yellow layer covering the white layer, this prompted me to change the recipe in the second week: Chinese absinthe (50 g) + Chinese mugwort (50 g) + Yu Ping Feng San, for five days, with the same moxibustion and foot bath recommendations.

He then confirmed to me that he was cured. Nevertheless, I still noticed a small yellow layer on his tongue, so I advised him to drink Chinese absinthe infusion (50 g) for another five days, with the same foot bath recipe.

He called me back afterwards to tell me that not only was he cured, but that he had never felt better, so fit, and with a perfect sleep. He even told me that he had lost some weight and that he felt young, that life was beautiful! He was so happy that I still feel it as I write these lines.

8. Other Tips by Categories of Cold, Flu and Covid-19

In case of emergency, it is first necessary to treat the symptoms and determine through various tools (tongue, pulse, etc.) whether it is a cold or a hot or cold flu, in order to prepare the different treatments better (the same goes for Covid-19).

– If the origin is cold: the symptoms are on the Yin side, i.e. white palate, flu state with sensitivity to wind and cold, absence of perspiration, clear nasal discharge, cough with white mucus.
Recommendations :
   a) Grated ginger soup (two tablespoons) + one to two tablespoons full-bodied brown sugar. To be taken every morning on an empty stomach until the total disappearance of symptoms (like the following infusion, do not take after healing, unless recommended by a doctor).
   b) Dried mandarin peel (50 g) + dried licorice stick (10 g). This is an infusion, so it can as well be taken three times a day until the symptoms have completely disappeared.

– If the category of the disease is hot: the symptoms are on the Yang side, i.e. yellow and/or red palate, flu state with hyperthermia, sweating, dry nose or with thick yellow discharge, yellow or dry layer on the tongue

Recommendations :

a) Chinese turnip soup (Bai Luo Bo) + honey (to be dosed according to preference) ;

b) Apple soup + pear (Chinese or Japanese pear) + banana.

Dice them and boil them with white cane (or crystal) sugar, as it has Yin energy.

Always dice to facilitate cooking and to benefit from the maximum of properties.

We do not give any proportions or quantities, as it is up to each person to choose according to his or her taste. It can be a dessert or even a complete meal; there is no strict rule. Indeed, for these last recipes, we are no longer addressing treatments as recommended by traditional Chinese medicine, but rather nutritional advice, which is nevertheless a decisive factor in the healing process. This is the topic of the next chapter.

Dried licorice sticks and infusion

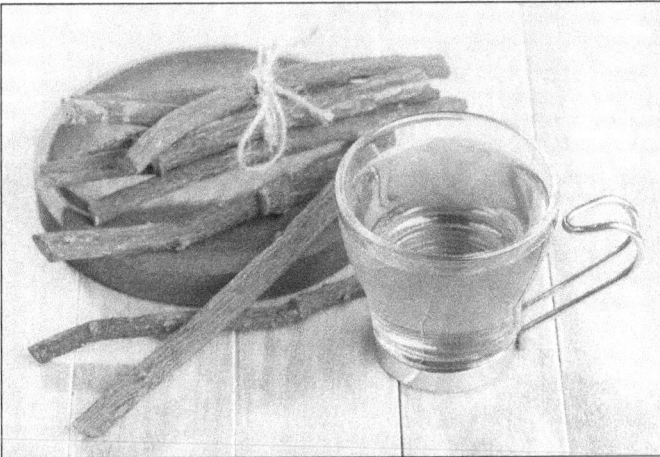

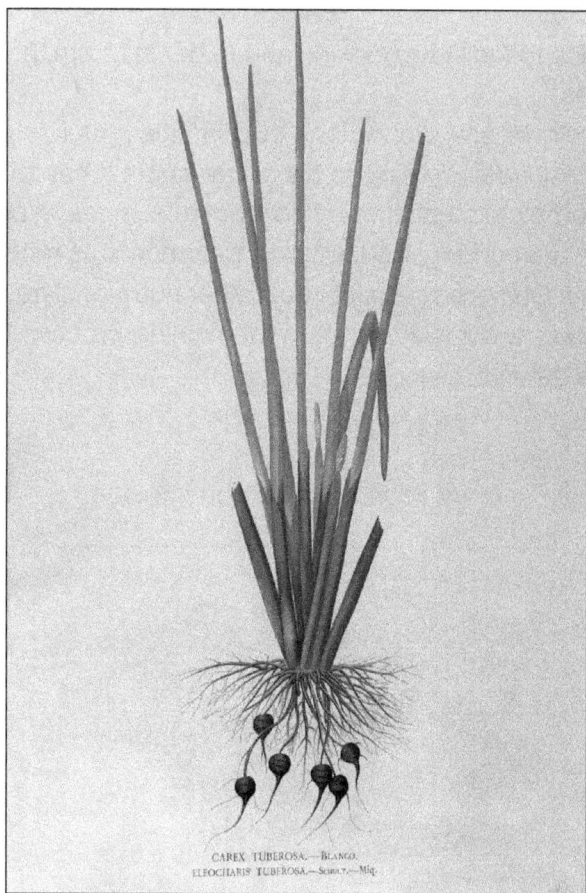

CAREX TUBEROSA.—BLANCO.
ELEOCHARIS TUBEROSA.—Schult.—Miq.

The water chestnut

Chapter VI

Suggested Accompaniments

During this period, I was often asked whether there were foods to be consumed as a priority for our health, in addition to specific recipes to treat symptoms,. This is the case, as my regular patients and students know.

As this is "recommended food" and not "treatment," there is, in most cases presented in this chapter, no indication of proportions or quantities: it is up to each person to choose according to what he/she likes. This notion is also vital in our practice because if the body takes pleasure, it generates positive energy, which increases the effectiveness of the treatment.

Consequently, I have communicated lists of products, out of which each person can pick and choose according to their taste, culinary tradition, seasonality and availability of ingredients.

Here are some examples to know in case of a virus, but also in everyday life, especially to strengthen our immune system.

1. Nutrition and Cooking

The following dishes and foods are recommended in cases of Covid-19, cough, cold, flu, fever:

– black mushroom soup: black is the color of the kidneys and cleanses the pulmonary tract;

– millet broth: it boosts the body's energy and stimulates the immune system;

– ginkgo: effective for its antibacterial virtues, cleanses the pulmonary tracts, calms coughs and reduces mucus (it is more practical to consume it in capsules, on the basis of seven per day);

– white radish: it purifies the lungs, soothes coughs, reduces throat pain, deflates the stomach, reduces mucus;

– dried lily flowers: they are eaten as vegetables or dried mushrooms, sautéed, in a soup, in a pot. They give Yin energy, stimulate blood circulation, relax and remove nervousness;

– pork tenderloin: this part next to the animal's kidneys boosts the energy of ours. Moreover, unlike other meats, pork is neutral in energy, i.e. balanced in Yin and Yang, so it is to be preferred in case of illness, after childbirth or an operation, and in case of a fall in vitality, in general.

2. More Infusions

We have already presented several recipes, but here are some other ones to vary the pleasures according to the availability of ingredients. The possibilities of infusion being almost infinite, we have chosen them according to their relation to the symptoms of Covid-19 and other lung infections :

– Chenpi 50 g + liquorice 20 g + tangerine fiber 10 g: calms cough, removes mucus, improves bronchitis and asthma;

– mulberry leaves (preferably autumn mulberry, as this is the season for the lungs) + apricot kernels: useful for lung cleansing; the almond is more effective, but it must be boiled first, as it is difficult to digest;

– dried yellow chrysanthemum flowers + dried liquorice: calms the Yang cough and relaxes the body;

– dried white hibiscus flowers + mint leaves (fresh or dried) + dried Osmanthus flowers + dried jasmine flowers: calms cough, removes mucus and increases lung energy.

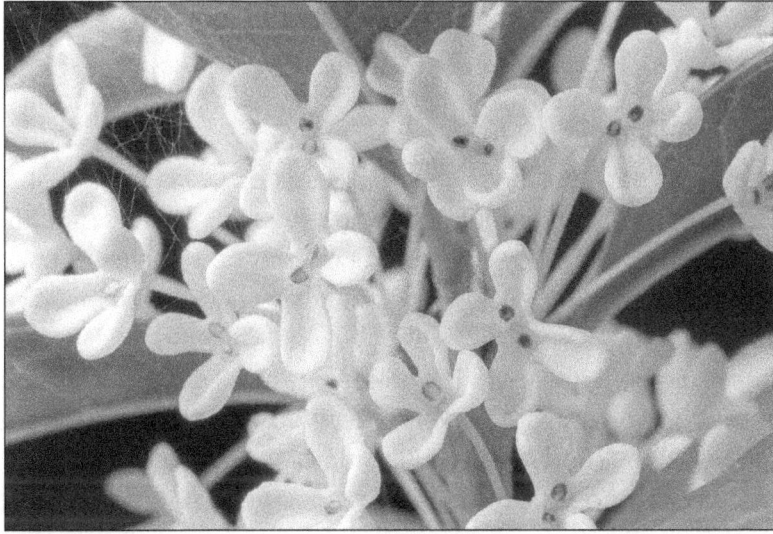

Osmanthus flowers

Banned!

Foods not recommended while treating Covid-19, the flu, a cold:
– shellfish and seafood, cold drinks, because they prevent the evacuation of mucus and thicken it, being mostly Yin energy.
– fat foods disrupt the drop in temperature, make digestion more difficult.
– spicy foods, milk, tea, coffee, tobacco, alcohol (non-exhaustive list), as they can alter the effectiveness of care and worsen symptoms.
As a general principle, it is better to eat lightly when taking treatment and, in any case, to follow your doctor's recommendations.

3. Clementine or Orange Fiber

It is very effective in purifying blockages of circulation in the airways and lungs.

When you eat an orange or a clementine, get into the habit of consuming the fiber, not just drinking the juice, as it helps to fight flu symptoms, etc. They are also recommended against smoking, which causes a Yin deficiency in the lungs and causes mucus to build up.

Here is a recent case: Mr. T. smoked one pack a day and coughed daily, especially at night, which prevented him from sleeping and weakened him. There was a suspicion of Covid-19 when he came to me. My diagnosis allowed me to reassure him. I recommended to drink twice a day for five days the composition mulberry branch or root + apricot kernel + ginseng + medlar leaves + *Ophiopogon japonicus* + Fritillaria, with the proportions of twenty grams for each plant, and, if possible, to stop smoking.

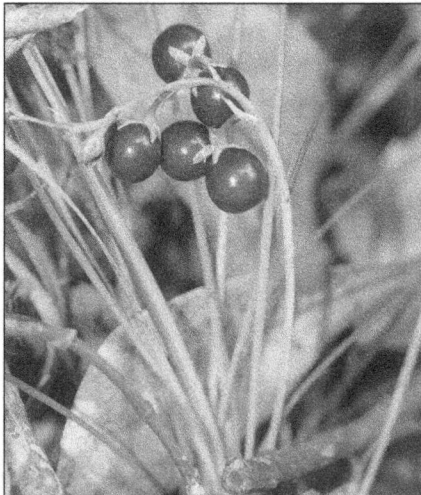

Ophiopogon japonicus

As he told me he found a bag of dried mandarin fibers in a drawer, given to him by his mother on her last trip to China, precisely to improve his lung problems linked to his addiction, I advised him to add fifteen grams to the recipe.

Five days later, he confirmed to me that the cough was almost definitely gone.

Afterwards, I suggested that he should adopt good eating habits, especially eating fruits like apples. As for quitting smoking, it's up to him. Traditional Chinese medicine actually offers solutions to help after the decision.

4. The Apple

Regular consumption improves heart and lung functions, which reduces the risk of asthma and pneumonia, promotes detoxification of the body, especially the lungs, and reduces the occurrence of coughs and sputum because they contain pectin and antioxidants.

Eating apples is therefore particularly recommended in case of symptoms of Covid-19 and other viruses.

The majority of the different varieties are neutral in nature, except for green apples, which are slightly Yin. In the case of Covid-19 flu, choose preferably red and/or yellow apples: red, they are intended for the heart and liver; yellow, for the spleen; as for the white part inside, it is intended for the lungs. An apple after each meal is excellent in case of symptoms.

After fries, doughnuts, chips, nuggets, I also recommend eating an apple, which I do myself or with my children, to get rid of the nervousness generated by these foods and the feeling of dryness in the throat, while developing a "degreasing" effect.

I have shared this suggestion with different groups, especially mothers, who can't stop their children from eating doughnuts and nuggets. They tell me that they now agree to it, but only on the condition that they eat an apple after the meal, which is accepted by the family. More than a dozen of them have thanked me for this simple and easy trick because they find their children less nervous. For four of them with bright red lips (a sign of nervousness in TCM), who were starting to cough, it only took three apples a day to solve the problem. I even recommended for the third apple, the one after dinner, to slice it and sprinkle it lightly with licorice powder to remove the cough. Of the four children, the cough and the feeling of nervousness disappeared the very next day in one case, after two dinners for two of them, and in three evenings for the fourth. Of course, there was a condition: do not consume doughnuts during this period.

5. Black and White Sesame

As presented in Chapter II, traditional Chinese medicine has a particular color for each organ: black for the kidneys and white for the lungs. Sesame is therefore recommended in cases of lung infection and/or kidney problems.

Both types of sesame seeds are also valuable because, among other benefits, they are rich in calcium: one single grain is equivalent to a glass of milk. This is all the more important in China as a large part of the population is intolerant to cow milk. However, it is important to chew the grains well, otherwise, the body cannot absorb all their properties.

Sesame (white or black) promotes digestion and also helps to fight constipation.

Finally, it is an asset for beauty because it goes into the lungs and kidneys, which manage the skin, nails and hair.

6. Other Benefits

– Both in the groups and with my patients, I recommend eating buckwheat seeds at least once a week, possibly in the form of noodles, to help digestion and facilitate the evacuation of what is troublesome. The majority of them have followed this advice, which is becoming a habit, even if it is not a traditional diet in China. However, buckwheat is present in the treatises of traditional Chinese medicine.

– Grapefruit juice or youzu + honey = cleansing of the respiratory tract.

– Mint infusion + honey = cleansing of the respiratory tract.

Especially in spring, with symptoms such as pollen allergies, coughing, itchy or dry throat, etc. these infusions are generally effective, as shown by the exchanges in the groups where I have recommended them.

Be sure to choose quality honey, one that really comes from hives.

7. Cinnamon

This spice is ideal for winter ailments: colds, coughs, flu and other viruses, including Covid-19. Indeed, due to its antioxidant properties, its high minerals and vitamins content, it strengthens and stimulates the immune system, has antiviral and antimicrobial properties, relieves digestion problems and intervenes naturally on type 2 diabetes.

I have had two positive feedbacks from people who have used it for heartburn, but no examples of its effects against Covid-19 because it was mixed with other ingredients and recipes.

8. Garlic + Thai Chives

This soup is very useful to remove fever and detoxify the organs. It is a traditional recipe from Chinese medicine, found in many ancient medical treatises. Still, I have no feedback on its effectiveness, as I recommended my grandmother's recipe, which adds ginger (seen in *Chapter V*).

9. The Coriander

It is a slightly warm plant (Yang).
Properties: purifies the pulmonary and respiratory tracts, facilitates by sweating the evacuation of blockages and what is negative, lowers fever, throat pain, helps digestion, reduces swelling of the stomach, stops diarrhea, has antibacterial properties, reduces fatigue.

Coriander is sometimes consumed to fight anxiety and promote sleep.

It is therefore recommended in case of symptoms related to Covid-19, flu, colds, rheumatism.

10. Pi Shu (Spleen) and Shen Shu (Kidneys) Points

After curing Covid-19, flu, colds, etc., it is essential to strengthen the immune system in order to regain your energy as quickly as possible. According to traditional Chinese medicine, the kidneys represent the energy before birth, and the spleen represents the energy after birth, so if these two organs are stimulated, all the energy of the body is stimulated. Consequently, moxibustion is particularly indicated in the following two points:

– Pi Shu (脾俞), international reference BL20
It is located on the back, 1.5 cun's distance to the left and right, at the bottom of the eleventh vertebra.

– Shen Shu (肾俞), international reference BL23
It is located on the back, 1.5 cun's distance to the left and right below the second vertebra of the lumbar spine.

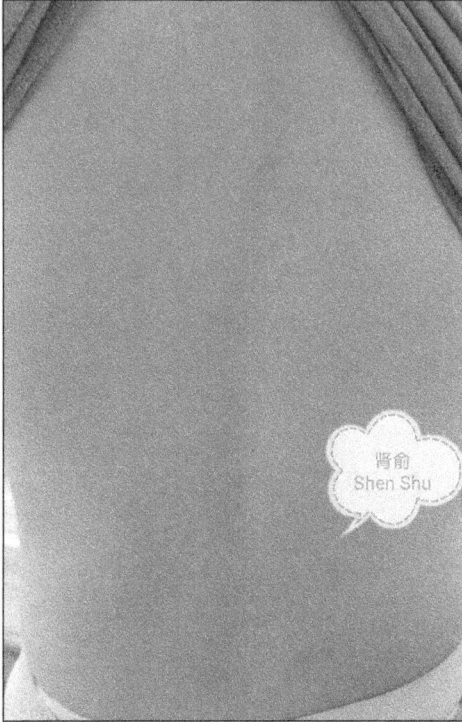

A Little Exercise to Finish up!
The Eight Pieces of Brocades or Ba Duan Jin (八段锦)

Ba Duan Jin is included in medical university curricula and has been promoted nationally since 2003 by the State General Administration of Sport as a "Health Qigong."

It is a "fitness" method invented in ancient China by General Yue Fei (1103-1142) to improve the health and physical condition of his soldiers. Originally, it consisted of twelve body movements, including a breathing technique, which was later reduced to eight. The meaning of the name is uncertain, but it evokes the rich fabrics worn by the dignitaries, which meant that during practice the movements had to be continuous and supple, like silk. Before executing them, it is advisable to practice some muscular awakening exercises and to stretch.

The eight postures are practiced in sequence, either sitting or standing.

On the drawings of the original version of General Yue Fei, they each have an evocative name that can be translated as follows:

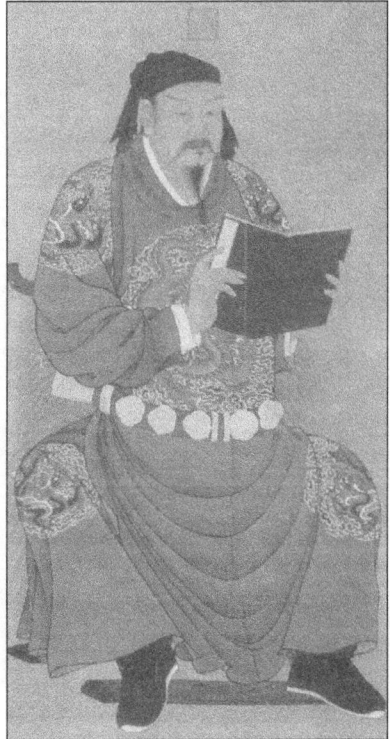

111

1. *Liang shou tuo tian li san jiao* (两手托天理三焦), "Supporting the sky with hands takes care of the triple heater."
This movement concerns three important regions of the body, i.e. above the diaphragm, between the diaphragm and the navel, between the navel and the pubis. This exercise regulates the Qi and promotes breathing, digestion and elimination.

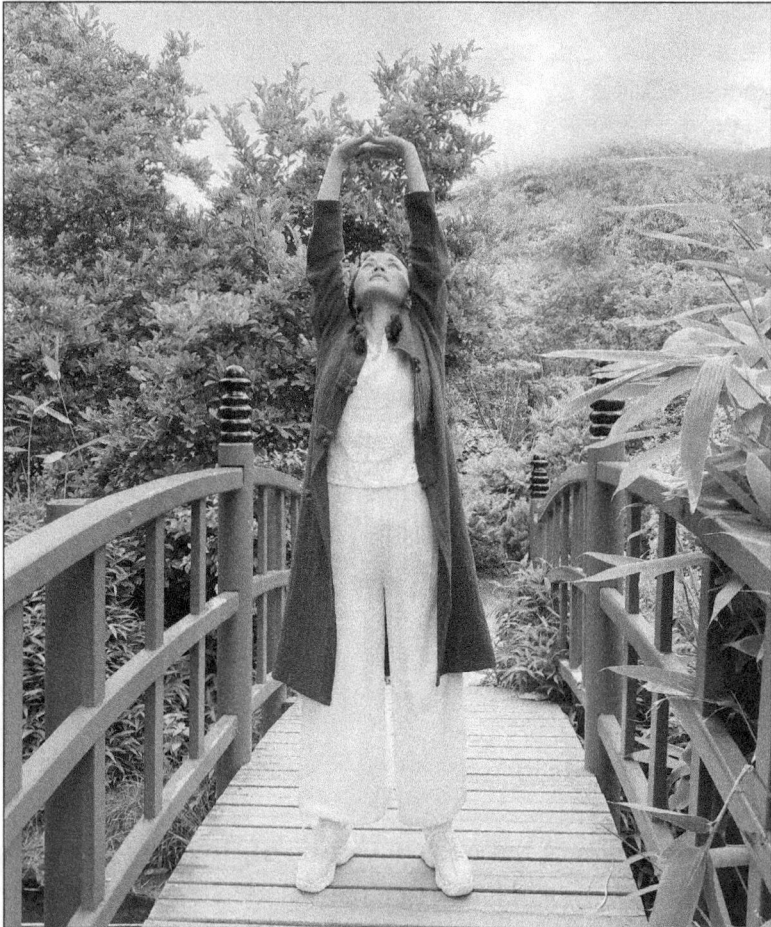

2. *Zuo you kai gong si she diao* (左右开弓似射雕), "band the bow right and left and aim at the eagle" (do on each side).
It facilitates circulation in the body and strengthens the Qi of the heart and lungs.

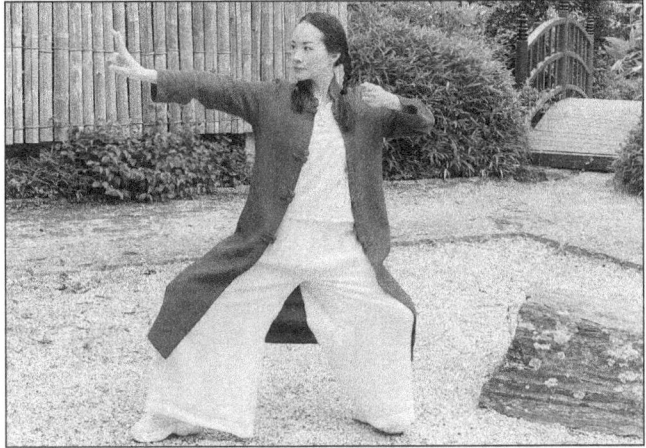

3. *Tiao li pi wei xu dan ju* (调理脾胃须单举), "Stimulate the spleen and stomach with a single gesture."
This movement stimulates the circulation of energy in the spleen, stomach and liver.

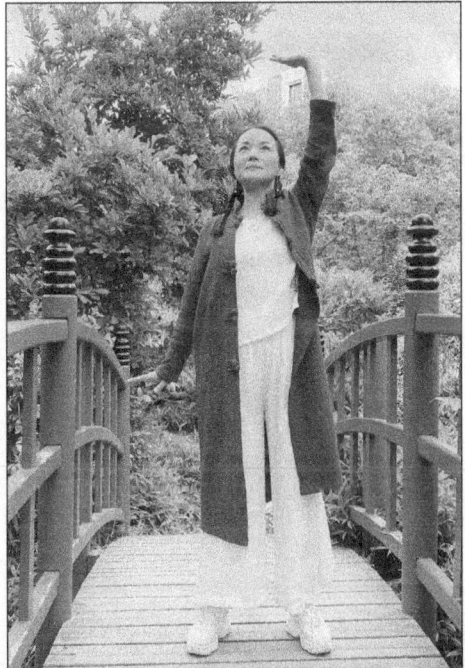

4. *Wu lao qi shang xiang hou qiao* (五劳七伤向后瞧), "looking back to prevent the five diseases and seven injuries."

The five diseases concern the five organs: heart, lungs, liver, kidneys and spleen, while "the seven injuries" represent the seven emotions, which we must learn to manage: anger, joy, sadness, fear, worry, obsession. Otherwise, their excess or inhibition is a source of disease, affecting the organs.

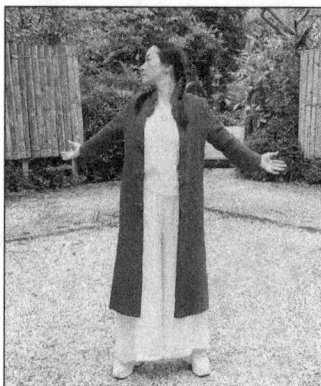

5. *Yao tou bai wei qu xinhuo* (摇头摆尾去心火), "shake your head and shake your tail to calm the fire of the heart."

This movement stimulates the lungs and reduces the "fire" of the heart if it is excessive.

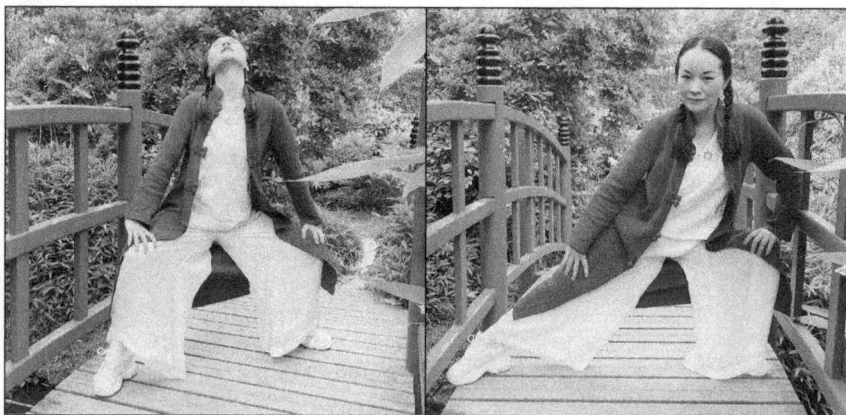

6. *Liang shou pan zu gu shen yao* (两手攀足固肾腰), "grabbing the toes to strengthen the kidneys."
Movement that invigorates the kidneys, as the name indicates.

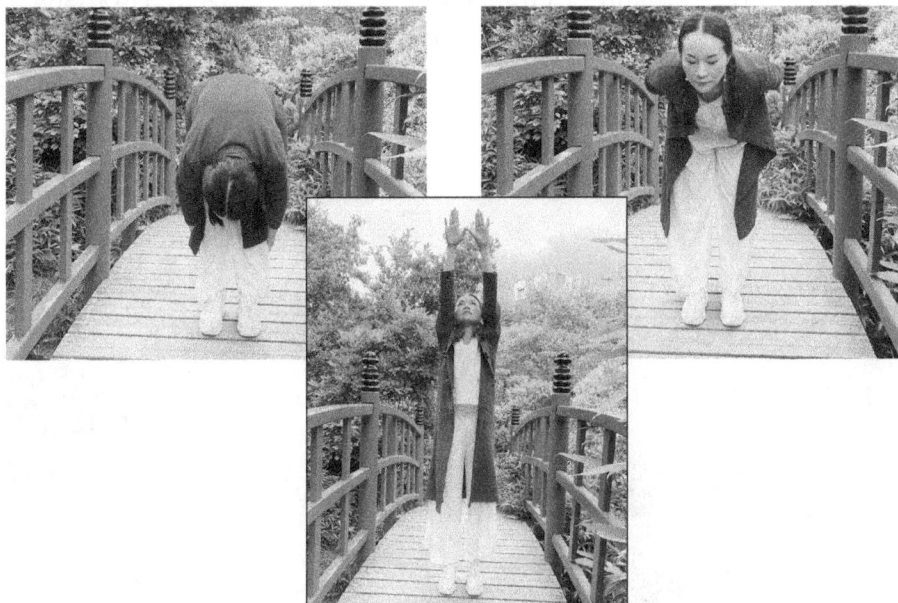

7. *Cuan quan numu zeng qili* (攒拳怒目增气力), "clenching fists with eyes of fire to increase physical strength."
The exercise that coordinates concentration, strength and vital breath. It stimulates the energy of the liver and removes its blockages, including stress, nervousness and anxiety, which damage this organ.

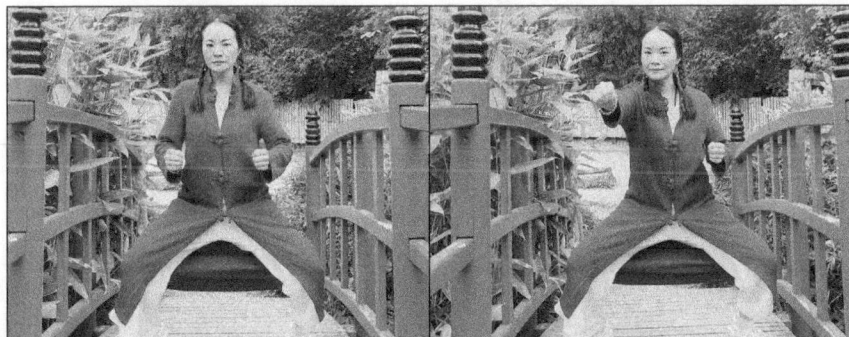

8. *Bei hou qi dian bai bing xiao* (背后七颠百病消), "Gently lift and let go the heels seven times to treat disease."
This movement activates the meridians of the feet, re-aligns the lumbar vertebrae and promotes the circulation of Qi in all organs from the kidneys. It is important to finish with this exercise, as it serves as a closure to regain all the energy in serenity. Accompany it with a gesture of gratitude.

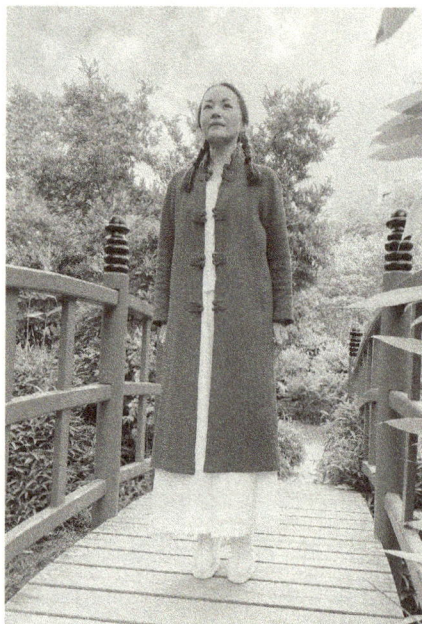

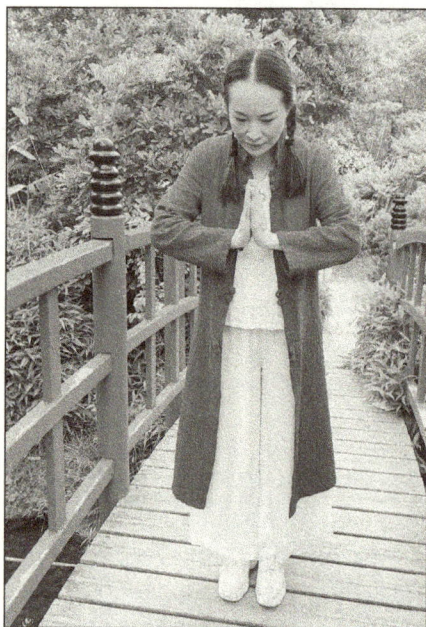

Ba Duan Jin is a gentle and light practice that helps to stimulate and preserve energy in the body, to help us find the Yin and Yang balance, not only in times of confinement but also throughout the rest of the year.

Conclusion

The traditional Chinese medicine and its various techniques have shown that Covid-19 and other viruses are not unbeatable, quite the contrary: we have all experienced it together during this difficult period in France, Italy, China.

Other epidemics will occur, if only seasonal flu, or even Covid-19 again. In order to better resist them, we must not just wait for them to come, but stimulate prevention, by progressively adopting the precepts and habits recommended by TCM, without forcing, simply by taking advantage of its benefits, through knowledge of food, by listening to our bodies, by knowing how to communicate with them, by using the soft method, which can become a daily practice and embellish our lives.

So strengthen your immune system,

Liberate your energy,

And be well!

Appendix 1

Diagnosis of the Tongue

We have seen its importance in the previous pages, particularly during a lockout and for remote care. Indeed, in Chinese medicine, this tool is crucial to detect health problems in a patient. There are two types of diagnosis: appearance and surface layer.

1) Appearance of the tongue:
   – color: pink, pale, red, dark red or crimson, purplish red;
   – shape: bloated, thin, cracked, with tooth marks, spiky;
   – condition: hard, weak, floating, trembling, deviated.
For example, a patient who has had a stroke will have a rather trembling tongue.

2) Layer of the tongue:
   – color: white, yellow, gray, black;
   – shape: thick, moist, dry, plastered and exfoliated.

It is possible to appreciate the level of energy, increasing or weakened, by looking at the state of the tongue. For example, a pink color indicates strong energy and good blood circulation, while a pale tongue indicates insufficient energy and blood, a slight white layer with a shine indicates strong stomach energy, a tongue without a layer but cracked indicates the opposite, i.e. insufficient stomach Yin energy.

Observing the tongue helps to locate the origin of the disease: if the color is red, the disease is related to energy; dark red, it affects the blood; a thin layer indicates that the origin of the disease is shallow; thick, that the disease is inside the body.

The tongue is also used to distinguish the nature of the disease. If there are petechiae[17] it is blood stasis. If it is bloated, it can be seen as a phlegm deficit or energy deficiency. The yellow layer comes mainly from excess heat, and the bloated layer is caused by phlegm, moisture and food accumulation.

The tongue can also be used to determine the course of the disease. For example, if the surface changes from white to yellow, then from yellow to grey or black, it means that the disease is transmuting from the surface to the inside, from cold to warm, which marks the worsening of the disease. When the layer of the tongue becomes thinner, it means that the disease is going away.

Here is a summarized presentation of several types of tongue appearances and layers in everyday life:

– Tongue Appearance

1. Pink, thin white layer: good health and good Yin and Yang balance.

2. Cracked: lack of basic Yin, like dry and cracked earth. Cracks are visible on the layer of the tongue in varying amounts and depths and in various shapes.

3. With tooth marks: this is a sign of excess moisture.

4. Lumpy and bloated: weakened Yang body energy and moisture.

– Tongue Layer

1. Thin and white: it indicates good health and a good Yin and Yang balance, which corresponds to a normal situation. In case of illness, the thin layer means that the disease remains on the surface and has not penetrated the body.

1. Thin with a slight white layer: superficial cold.

2. White and thick: combination of coldness and humidity.

3. White, slippery and viscous: presence of phlegm in the body or moisture trapped in the spleen.

---

17. Small red to purplish skin spot.

4. Yellow, very viscous, as if covered with a layer of yellow paint. The combination of heat and humidity forms the yellow paste layer. The yellow color indicates warmth and accumulation of negative Yin energy, signs of overfeeding and indigestion.

5. Greyish: the disease is deteriorating, attacking the body's organs from the outside in.

6. Black: transformed from the yellow or grey layer, it indicates that the disease is extremely serious. The black, dry surface is caused by heat and extreme Yin deficiency. The dry black tip of the tongue indicates that the heart is in excess of Yang energy. A black, slippery layer indicates that the Yang is extremely weakened and the Yin is extremely cold.

The correspondence of the tongue with the internal organs of the body:
– tip of the tongue: heart and lungs;
– middle: spleen and stomach;
– left border: liver;
– right border: gallbladder;
– root: kidneys.

Diagnosis With the Tongue

There's an old Chinese saying:

The pulse may lie, but the tongue tells the truth.

In traditional medicine, the condition of the tongue's layer is a signal sent by the body. The elders used their wisdom to dissect the tongue layer, leaving us with an incomparable and valuable identification pattern for future generations of doctors and their patients.

Appendix 2

Some Specific Words From Traditional Chinese Medicine Related to Covid-19

The term Covid-19 does not, of course, exist in traditional Chinese medicine, but here are the themes that allow us to understand its symptoms and the treatments to apply:

传统中医 (Zhongyi), TCM (Traditional Chinese Medicine)
风 (Fēng), Wind
风热 (Fēng Rè), Warm Wind / Warm Wind
风寒 (Fēng Hán), Cold wind
风湿 (Fēng Shī), Wet wind
风燥 (Fēng Zào), Dry Wind
八纲 (Bā Gāng), Eight Principles (of diagnosis)
表里 (Biāo/Li) Area/Depth
辨证论治 (Biàn Zhèng Lùn Zhì), Differential Diagnosis of Symptoms
病因 (Bîng Yīn), Etiology[18] of diseases
症状 (Zhèng Zhuàng), Symptom
湿热 (Shī Rè), Moisture-heat infringement
卫气 (Wei Qi), Protection / Defence Layer
湿 (Shī), Humidity
温病 (Wēn Bîng), Warm disease
湿温 (Shī Wen), Wet and Warm Disease
疫病 (Yî Bîng) /疫疬(Yî Lî), Epidemic disease
温疫 (Wēn Yî), Warm epidemic disease

18. In medicine, etiology (or etiopathogeny) is the study of the causes and factors of a disease. The term is also used in psychiatry and psychology to study the causes of mental illness. Etiology defines the origin of a disease according to signs or symptoms, i.e. in the jargon of its semiological manifestations. "Source: Wikipedia.

疟疾 (Nüè Ji), Malaria

痰饮 (Tán Yīn), Mucositis

邪 (or 邪气) Xié (or Xié Qî), Perversity

伏邪气 (or 伏气)Fú Xié Qî (or Fú Qî), Latent Perversity

虚 (Xu), Impairment (or Void)

恐 (Kǒng), Fear

伤寒 (Shāng Hán), Typhoid Fever / Cold Stroke.

Table of content

Table of boxes

Photo Credits

www.ingramcontent.com/pod-product-compliance
Lightning Source LLC
Chambersburg PA
CBHW030253030426
42336CB00009B/371